THE DR. SEBI HEALING BIBLE
| 20 IN 1 |

The Ultimate Guide to Knowing ALL of Dr. Sebi's Studies on Common Diseases, the Alkaline Diet, and the Non-Toxic Lifestyle.
A Mind-Opening Book.

Kelly Outtara

Table of Contents

Book 1: The Alkaline Lifestyle: Dr. Sebi's Guide to Optimal Health and Wellness 1

    Introduction to the Alkaline Lifestyle 2

    Dr. Sebi's Nutritional Philosophy 6

    Implementing the Alkaline Diet 10

    Alkaline Lifestyle for Specific Health Goals 14

    Beyond Diet: Embracing a Holistic Alkaline Lifestyle 18

Book 2: Healing Naturally: Dr. Sebi's Approach to Curing Stds 20

    Understanding Sexually Transmitted Diseases (STDS) 21

    Herbal Remedies for STDS 25

    Alkaline Diet and STDS 29

    Holistic Approaches to Long-Term Healing 31

Book 3: Herpes No More: Dr. Sebi's Natural Remedies for Herpes 33

    Understanding Herpes: Types and Symptoms 34

    Dr. Sebi's Herbal Recommendations for Herpes 37

    Adopting an Alkaline Diet for Herpes Management 40

Book 4: HIV-Free Living: Dr. Sebi's Holistic Solutions for HIV 44

    Understanding HIV: Transmission and Progression 45

    Dr. Sebi's Herbal Support for HIV 47

    The Alkaline Diet for HIV Management 49

    Embracing Positivity and Hope: Living Fully with HIV 50

Book 5: Defeating Diabetes: Dr. Sebi's Path to Reversing Diabetes Naturally ... 52

    Understanding Diabetes: Types and Risk Factors 53

    Dr. Sebi's Herbal Remedies for Diabetes 56

The Alkaline Diet for Diabetes Control 59

Exercise and Diabetes Management 61

Living Well with Diabetes: Empowering a Healthy Lifestyle 64

Book 6: Lupus Unraveled: Dr. Sebi's Natural Treatment for Lupus 69

Understanding Lupus: Types and Symptoms 70

Dr. Sebi's Herbal Recommendations for Lupus 73

Adopting an Alkaline Diet for Lupus Management 76

Managing Emotional Wellbeing with Lupus 79

Thriving with Lupus: Embracing a Life Beyond the Diagnosis 79

Book 7: Healthy Hair, Naturally: Dr. Sebi's Guide to Preventing Hair Loss ... 84

Understanding Hair Loss: Causes and Types 85

Dr. Sebi's Herbal Remedies for Hair Loss 88

The Alkaline Diet for Healthy Hair 91

Hair Care Practices for Preventing Hair Loss 94

Embracing Natural Beauty: Empowering Hair Care Choices 98

Book 8: Cancer-Free Living: Dr. Sebi's Approach to Fighting Cancer Holistically ... 101

Understanding Cancer: Causes and Risk Factors 102

Dr. Sebi's Herbal Support for Cancer Patients 106

The Alkaline Diet for Cancer Management 109

Holistic Lifestyle Strategies for Cancer Prevention 111

Thriving Beyond Cancer: Embracing a Life of Healing 113

Book 9: Breaking Free from Kidney Stones: Dr. Sebi's Natural Kidney Stone Solutions ... 118

Kidney Stones: Causes and Symptoms 119

Dr. Sebi's Herbal Remedies for Kidney Stones 122

The Alkaline Diet for Kidney Stone Prevention 126

Embracing Kidney Health: Empowering a Stone-Free Life.......................... 129

Book 10: Heart Health Unleashed: Dr. Sebi's Guide to a Healthy Heart.............. 131

Heart Disease: Risk Factors and Prevention.. 132

Dr. Sebi's Herbal Support for Heart Health 137

The Alkaline Diet for a Strong Heart 143

Exercise and Lifestyle for Cardiovascular Health.. 148

Book 11: Easing Arthritis: Dr. Sebi's Natural Remedies for Arthritis 154

Understanding Arthritis: Types and Symptoms 155

Dr. Sebi's Herbal Recommendations for Arthritis 161

The Alkaline Diet for Arthritis Relief... 165

Lifestyle Practices for Arthritis Management.. 170

Living Comfortably with Arthritis: Empowering a Pain-Free Life 176

Book 12: Clear Skin Naturally: Dr. Sebi's Approach to Radiant Skin 182

Skin Health: Common Skin Issues and Causes 183

Dr. Sebi's Herbal Support for Healthy Skin... 186

The Alkaline Diet for Glowing Skin 190

Embracing Skin Confidence: Nurturing Your True Beauty 194

Book 13: Beating High Blood Pressure: Dr. Sebi's Guide to Hypertension Management......... 200

Understanding Hypertension: Causes and Risk Factors............................... 201

Dr. Sebi's Herbal Remedies for High Blood Pressure 206

The Alkaline Diet for Blood Pressure Control.. 210

Lifestyle Strategies for Hypertension Management 214

Book 14: Detoxify Your Body: Dr. Sebi's Cleansing and Detoxification Methods..................... 219

The Importance of Detoxification for Health 220

Dr. Sebi's Herbal Detox Remedies 224

The Alkaline Diet for Detoxification 228

Book 15: Boosting Immune Power: Dr. Sebi's Natural Solutions for a Strong Immune System 232

Understanding the Immune System and its Functions 233

Dr. Sebi's Immune-Enhancing Herbs and Practices.. 238

The Alkaline Diet for Optimal Immune Function 243

Lifestyle Strategies to Support Immunity.. 248

Book 16: Restoring Digestive Health: Dr. Sebi's Remedies for a Happy Gut 254

Gut Health: Common Digestive Issues and Causes.. 255

Dr. Sebi's Herbal Support for Digestive Health... 260

The Alkaline Diet for a Balanced Gut 265

Lifestyle Practices for Digestive Wellness 270

Book 17: Beating Insomnia Naturally: Dr. Sebi's Guide to Restful Sleep.................... 272

Understanding Insomnia: Causes and Symptoms.. 273

Dr. Sebi's Herbal Recommendations for Better Sleep 277

Lifestyle Habits for Promoting Restful Sleep 281

Book 18: Mental Clarity Unleashed: Dr. Sebi's Path to Cognitive Health.................... 284

Cognitive Health: Enhancing Memory and Focus 285

Dr. Sebi's Herbal Remedies for Brain Health 287

The Alkaline Diet for Cognitive Enhancement 290

Lifestyle Practices for Optimal Brain Function 292

Book 19: Joint Freedom: Dr. Sebi's Natural Solutions for Joint Health 295

Joint Health: Common Issues and Causes.. 296

Dr. Sebi's Herbal Support for Healthy Joints 297

The Alkaline Diet for Joint Comfort 300

Lifestyle Strategies for Joint Flexibility 302

Embracing Active Living: A Path to Pain-Free Joints 304

Book 20: Dr. Sebi's Alkaline Kitchen: Mouthwatering Plant-Based Recipes 307

Dr. Sebi's Alkaline Breakfast Creations 308

Wholesome Alkaline Lunch Delights 310

Nourishing Alkaline Snacks and Desserts 312

Satisfying Alkaline Dinner Delicacies 314

Book 1: The Alkaline Lifestyle: Dr. Sebi's Guide to Optimal Health and Wellness

Introduction to the Alkaline Lifestyle

The alkaline lifestyle is a holistic approach to health and well-being centered around maintaining the body's pH level in an alkaline state. It is based on the idea that consuming alkaline-forming foods and beverages can help neutralize acidity in the body, leading to improved health, increased energy levels, and a reduced risk of various health issues.

1. Understanding pH:

The pH scale measures the acidity or alkalinity of a substance and ranges from 0 to 14. A pH of 7 is considered neutral, below 7 is acidic, and above 7 is alkaline. The human body has a natural pH range between 7.35 and 7.45, which is slightly alkaline. However, due to various factors such as stress, poor diet, lack of exercise, and environmental toxins, our bodies can become more acidic, leading to potential health problems.

2. Acid-Alkaline Balance:

The alkaline lifestyle emphasizes the importance of maintaining an optimal acid-alkaline balance within the body. Proponents of this lifestyle argue that excess acidity can create an environment conducive to inflammation, weakened immune function, and chronic diseases. By consuming alkaline-forming foods, individuals aim to bring their pH back into balance and improve overall health.

3. Alkaline-Forming Foods:

Alkaline-forming foods are typically plant-based, nutrient-dense foods that help raise the body's pH levels. Some examples of alkaline-forming foods include:

- Fruits: Such as lemons, watermelons, avocados, and bananas.
- Vegetables: Like leafy greens (spinach, kale, lettuce), cucumbers, broccoli, and bell peppers.
- Nuts and Seeds: Almonds, chia seeds, and flaxseeds are good examples.
- Whole Grains: Quinoa, millet, and amaranth are considered alkaline-forming.
- Herbal Teas: Chamomile, peppermint, and ginger teas are alkaline-promoting beverages.

4. Acid-Forming Foods to Avoid:

In contrast to alkaline-forming foods, acid-forming foods are believed to contribute to higher acidity levels in the body. These foods are often associated with modern diets high in processed foods, sugars, and unhealthy fats. Some examples of acid-forming foods include:

- Processed Foods: Fast foods, packaged snacks, and pre-made meals.
- Sugar and Sweets: Soft drinks, candies, and desserts.
- Meat and Dairy: Beef, pork, chicken, and cow's milk products.
- Refined Grains: White bread, white rice, and pasta made from refined flour.
- Caffeine and Alcohol: Coffee, tea, and alcoholic beverages.

5. Benefits of the Alkaline Lifestyle:

Advocates of the alkaline lifestyle claim that adhering to an alkaline-promoting diet and incorporating other alkaline practices can provide numerous benefits, including:

- Increased Energy: Improved pH balance can lead to higher energy levels and reduced fatigue.
- Better Digestion: Alkaline-forming foods are often high in fiber, aiding digestion and promoting gut health.
- Weight Management: A balanced pH may support weight loss and maintenance efforts.
- Enhanced Immune Function: Alkaline environments may help the immune system function optimally.
- Reduced Inflammation: Lower acidity levels are believed to reduce inflammation in the body.
- Healthy Skin: Clearer, healthier skin is often attributed to an alkaline lifestyle.

6. The Alkaline Lifestyle Beyond Diet:

While nutrition plays a central role in the alkaline lifestyle, it extends beyond just food choices. Other aspects include:

- Hydration: Drinking alkaline water is encouraged to support pH balance.
- Stress Management: Stress reduction techniques, such as meditation and yoga, are recommended.

- Exercise: Regular physical activity helps maintain overall health and promotes a balanced pH.
- Sleep: Sufficient sleep is essential for the body's natural healing processes.

7. Alkaline Water:

Alkaline water is a key component of the alkaline lifestyle. It is water that has a higher pH level than regular tap water, typically ranging between 8 and 9.5. Proponents of alkaline water claim that it can help neutralize acid in the body and provide additional health benefits. Some methods of producing alkaline water include adding alkaline minerals like magnesium and calcium or using water ionizers to increase the pH.

8. pH Testing and Monitoring:

Maintaining an alkaline lifestyle involves being mindful of the body's pH levels. Regular pH testing of urine or saliva can help individuals monitor their acidity-alkalinity balance. pH test strips or pH meters are readily available for this purpose. These tests can be done at home and provide insights into how dietary and lifestyle choices may be affecting the body's pH.

9. Potential Drawbacks and Criticisms:

While the alkaline lifestyle has gained popularity, it is not without its criticisms and skeptics. Some concerns include:

- Limited Scientific Evidence: While certain aspects of the alkaline lifestyle have shown potential benefits in limited studies, more robust research is needed to fully validate its claims.
- Individual Variability: The body's pH levels are tightly regulated by various physiological mechanisms. Some experts argue that dietary changes have minimal impact on blood pH, which remains stable within its healthy range.
- Restrictive Nature: The alkaline diet can be restrictive, making it challenging for some individuals to adhere to in the long term.

10. Personalization and Flexibility:

As with any dietary approach, the alkaline lifestyle should be personalized to suit individual needs and preferences. It is essential to maintain a balanced and varied diet, incorporating a wide range of nutrient-dense foods. Some individuals may find it beneficial to follow the alkaline lifestyle more strictly, while others might opt for a more flexible approach.

11. Consulting a Healthcare Professional:

Before making any significant dietary or lifestyle changes, it is crucial to consult a qualified healthcare professional or a registered dietitian. They can provide personalized guidance based on an individual's health status, medical history, and specific goals.

12. Integrating the Alkaline Lifestyle:

Integrating the alkaline lifestyle into daily routines involves gradual and sustainable changes. Here are some steps to get started:

- Gradually increase the consumption of alkaline-forming foods, such as fresh fruits and vegetables.
- Reduce intake of acid-forming foods, especially processed and unhealthy choices.
- Stay well-hydrated by drinking alkaline water or water with a slightly higher pH.
- Engage in regular physical activity to support overall health and pH balance.
- Practice stress-reduction techniques like mindfulness, meditation, or yoga.

Dr. Sebi's Nutritional Philosophy

Dr. Sebi, born Alfredo Darrington Bowman (1933-2016), was a self-proclaimed herbalist, natural healer, and holistic health advocate. He gained popularity for his claims of being able to cure various health conditions through his unique nutritional approach. Dr. Sebi's nutritional philosophy revolves around the concept of "electric" or "alkaline" foods, which he believed could detoxify and heal the body.

1. The Concept of Electric Foods:

Dr. Sebi's nutritional philosophy is centered on the concept of "electric" or "alkaline" foods. According to him, electric foods are those that are naturally found in nature, have a high pH, and are rich in minerals. These foods are believed to possess inherent healing properties, as they can help the body maintain an alkaline state and remove toxins.

2. The Alkaline Diet:

Dr. Sebi's nutritional recommendations largely align with an alkaline diet, which emphasizes consuming predominantly alkaline-forming foods to achieve an optimal pH balance in the body. The diet focuses on fresh, plant-based foods, and minimizes the consumption of acid-forming foods, processed foods, and animal products.

3. Approved Foods:

Dr. Sebi categorized foods into three groups:

- **Electric Foods:** These are the foundation of his nutritional philosophy and include vegetables, fruits, grains, nuts, and seeds. Examples of electric foods include leafy greens, avocados, berries, quinoa, and raw almonds.
- **Neutral Foods:** This category includes some starchy vegetables and certain grains, such as sweet potatoes, yams, and certain types of rice. These foods were considered acceptable but not as beneficial as electric foods.
- **Acidic Foods:** Acidic foods are discouraged in Dr. Sebi's diet. These include most meats, dairy products, refined sugars, processed foods, and artificial additives.

4. Elimination of Hybrid Foods:

Dr. Sebi's philosophy also included avoiding hybrid foods, which he believed were unnatural and harmful to the body. Hybrid foods are the result of crossbreeding different plant varieties to produce new cultivars. According to him, hybrid foods lack the natural electrical charge found in unadulterated, wild-grown foods, and they contribute to disease and toxicity.

5. Detoxification and Healing:

Dr. Sebi claimed that by adhering to his nutritional philosophy and consuming electric foods, the body could detoxify itself and heal from various ailments, including diabetes, high blood pressure, obesity, and even serious conditions like cancer and AIDS. He claimed that his approach could alkalize the body, create an inhospitable environment for disease-causing organisms, and promote overall health and longevity.

6. Controversy and Criticism:

Dr. Sebi's nutritional philosophy and healing claims have been highly controversial and met with skepticism from the medical and scientific communities. Many experts have criticized his ideas for lacking scientific evidence and for making bold claims without proper clinical studies. Additionally, some people have reported adverse effects from following his strict dietary guidelines.

7. Importance of Individualization:

As with any dietary approach, it's essential to recognize that individual responses to specific foods and dietary patterns can vary widely. While some individuals may report positive experiences with Dr. Sebi's nutritional philosophy, others may not find it suitable for their unique health needs and goals.

8. Lack of Scientific Evidence:

One of the main criticisms of Dr. Sebi's nutritional philosophy is the lack of scientific evidence to support his claims. While some aspects of an alkaline diet, such as consuming more fruits and vegetables, have been associated with health benefits in scientific studies, the extreme claims made by Dr. Sebi have not been substantiated by rigorous scientific research.

9. Restrictive Nature:

Dr. Sebi's dietary recommendations are highly restrictive, which can make it challenging for individuals to adhere to in the long term. Eliminating entire food groups, such as animal products and certain grains, may lead to nutritional deficiencies if not carefully balanced with appropriate substitutes.

10. Lack of Individualization:

Dr. Sebi's approach takes a one-size-fits-all approach to health, assuming that all individuals will benefit from the same strict dietary guidelines. However, nutritional needs can vary significantly from person to person based on factors such as age, gender, activity level, and health conditions.

11. Positive Aspects:

While Dr. Sebi's nutritional philosophy has been met with skepticism, some positive aspects can be found in his recommendations. For example:

- Promoting Whole Foods: Dr. Sebi encourages the consumption of whole, natural foods, particularly fruits and vegetables, which are rich in vitamins, minerals, and antioxidants.
- Plant-Based Emphasis: His approach advocates for a plant-based diet, which has been associated with numerous health benefits, including a reduced risk of chronic diseases like heart disease and certain cancers.
- Hydration: Dr. Sebi emphasizes the importance of staying hydrated and consuming alkaline water, which can be beneficial for overall health.

12. Personal Responsibility:

Individuals who choose to follow Dr. Sebi's nutritional philosophy or any alternative approach to health should take personal responsibility for their decisions. It is essential to remain informed, critically evaluate health claims, and consult with qualified healthcare professionals to ensure that dietary choices align with individual health needs.

13. Integrating Principles into a Balanced Diet:

Instead of following Dr. Sebi's philosophy rigidly, some individuals may choose to incorporate certain principles into their overall dietary pattern. For example:

- Prioritize plant-based foods: Increase the intake of fruits, vegetables, nuts, and seeds in the diet.
- Reduce processed foods: Minimize the consumption of processed and refined foods high in sugar, salt, and unhealthy fats.
- Stay hydrated: Consume an adequate amount of water daily to support hydration and overall health.
- Individualize the approach: Tailor dietary choices to meet individual health needs, preferences, and cultural considerations.

Implementing the Alkaline Diet

Implementing the alkaline diet involves making conscious and informed choices to consume predominantly alkaline-forming foods while reducing acidic foods. Here are more details on how to effectively incorporate the alkaline diet into your lifestyle:

1. Understanding pH Levels:

Before starting the alkaline diet, it's essential to have a basic understanding of pH levels and their impact on the body. As mentioned earlier, the pH scale ranges from 0 to 14, with 7 being neutral. A pH below 7 is acidic, and a pH above 7 is alkaline. The human body operates optimally within a slightly alkaline range of 7.35 to 7.45. The goal of the alkaline diet is to consume foods that support maintaining this pH balance.

2. Focus on Alkaline-Forming Foods:

The cornerstone of the alkaline diet is consuming alkaline-forming foods. These primarily include fresh fruits, vegetables, nuts, seeds, and some whole grains. Here are some examples of alkaline-forming foods:

- Fruits: Berries, apples, pears, watermelon, lemons, and limes.
- Vegetables: Leafy greens (spinach, kale, lettuce), broccoli, cucumbers, bell peppers, and zucchini.
- Nuts and Seeds: Almonds, chia seeds, flaxseeds, and pumpkin seeds.
- Whole Grains: Quinoa, millet, amaranth, and brown rice.
- Legumes: Lentils, chickpeas, and black beans.

3. Minimize Acid-Forming Foods:

To support the alkaline diet, it's crucial to minimize the consumption of acid-forming foods. These typically include processed foods, refined sugars, meats, dairy products, caffeine, and alcohol. Acidic foods may disrupt the body's pH balance and contribute to inflammation and other health issues.

4. Hydration with Alkaline Water:

Drinking alkaline water is a common practice within the alkaline lifestyle. Alkaline water has a higher pH level than regular tap water and is believed to aid in maintaining an alkaline environment in the body. You can purchase alkaline water or use water ionizers to make your own.

5. Meal Planning:

Meal planning is essential to ensure a well-balanced and alkaline-friendly diet. Focus on creating meals that incorporate a variety of alkaline-forming foods. A typical alkaline meal might include a large salad with leafy greens, cucumber, avocado, and lemon dressing, along with a quinoa and vegetable stir-fry.

6. Gradual Transition:

For some individuals, transitioning to the alkaline diet can be a significant change. Instead of making drastic changes overnight, consider gradually incorporating more alkaline foods into your existing diet while reducing acidic choices. This approach allows your taste buds and digestive system to adapt more easily.

7. Mindful Eating:

Practicing mindful eating can help you become more aware of how food affects your body and overall well-being. Pay attention to how different foods make you feel and listen to your body's signals. This can help you identify which foods are best for you and which ones you may need to limit.

8. Seek Professional Guidance:

If you have specific health concerns or medical conditions, it's essential to consult with a qualified healthcare professional or a registered dietitian before making significant changes to your diet. They can provide personalized advice and ensure that the alkaline diet aligns with your individual health needs.

9. Balance and Moderation:

While the alkaline diet emphasizes the consumption of alkaline-forming foods, it's crucial to remember the importance of balance and moderation. A well-rounded diet should include a variety of nutrients from different food groups to meet all nutritional needs.

10. Sample Alkaline Diet Plan:

To further illustrate how to implement the alkaline diet, here's a sample meal plan for a day:

Breakfast:

- Green Smoothie: Blend together spinach, kale, cucumber, banana, and a splash of almond milk. Add a tablespoon of chia seeds for extra nutrients.
- Alkaline Herbal Tea: Sip on a cup of peppermint or chamomile tea.

Mid-Morning Snack:

- Fresh Fruit Salad: Combine sliced watermelon, strawberries, and kiwi for a refreshing and alkalizing snack.

Lunch:

- Quinoa Salad: Prepare a quinoa salad with diced tomatoes, cucumbers, bell peppers, and black beans. Toss with a lemon-tahini dressing.
- Avocado Slices: Enjoy a few slices of avocado on the side.

Afternoon Snack:

- Raw Almonds: Snack on a handful of raw almonds for a dose of healthy fats and protein.

Dinner:

- Stir-Fry Veggies: Sauté a mix of broccoli, bell peppers, zucchini, and carrots in coconut oil with minced garlic and ginger.
- Baked Sweet Potato: Serve the stir-fry over a baked sweet potato for a satisfying and nutritious meal.

Evening Snack:

- Fresh Berries: Top off your day with a bowl of fresh berries like blueberries, raspberries, or blackberries.

11. Reading Food Labels:

When implementing the alkaline diet, it's essential to read food labels to identify acidic ingredients or additives. Avoid processed foods with preservatives, artificial colors, and high-fructose corn syrup. Instead, focus on whole, natural foods to maintain an alkaline-friendly diet.

12. Supportive Lifestyle Habits:

While diet is a critical component of the alkaline lifestyle, other lifestyle habits can also support overall health:

- Regular Exercise: Engage in physical activity that you enjoy, such as walking, jogging, yoga, or swimming, to support overall well-being.
- Stress Management: Incorporate stress-reduction techniques like meditation, deep breathing, or mindfulness to promote a balanced mind and body.
- Sufficient Sleep: Aim for 7-9 hours of quality sleep per night to allow the body to rest and rejuvenate.

13. Tracking Progress:

Keep track of how you feel and any changes you notice as you follow the alkaline diet. Some individuals report increased energy levels, improved digestion, and better skin health. Tracking your progress can help you stay motivated and make adjustments as needed.

14. Long-Term Approach:

The alkaline diet is not a quick-fix solution but a long-term approach to promoting health and well-being. Consistency and patience are essential to experience the potential benefits of the alkaline lifestyle.

Alkaline Lifestyle for Specific Health Goals

The alkaline lifestyle, with its focus on consuming alkaline-forming foods and promoting overall health, can be tailored to address specific health goals. Here are some examples of how the alkaline lifestyle can be implemented to support different health objectives:

1. Weight Management:

The alkaline diet, rich in nutrient-dense, low-calorie foods like fruits and vegetables, can be beneficial for weight management. These foods are often naturally lower in calories but high in fiber and water content, promoting a feeling of fullness and satiety. By adopting the alkaline lifestyle and reducing the intake of processed and high-calorie foods, individuals may find it easier to manage their weight and support healthy weight loss.

2. Digestive Health:

The alkaline lifestyle, with its emphasis on whole plant foods, can contribute to better digestive health. Fruits, vegetables, and whole grains are rich in fiber, which aids digestion and promotes regular bowel movements. Additionally, the diet avoids acidic and inflammatory foods that may contribute to digestive discomfort. Proper hydration with alkaline water can also support digestive health by preventing constipation and promoting hydration.

3. Heart Health:

An alkaline diet that is rich in fruits, vegetables, and whole grains can be beneficial for heart health. These foods are naturally low in cholesterol, saturated fats, and sodium, which are known risk factors for heart disease. The alkaline lifestyle also encourages the consumption of heart-healthy fats from sources like nuts and seeds, which can support cardiovascular health.

4. Diabetes Management:

The alkaline lifestyle may be beneficial for individuals with diabetes or those at risk of developing the condition. By focusing on low-glycemic, alkaline-forming foods, the diet can help regulate blood sugar levels. Reducing the intake of refined sugars and processed carbohydrates can contribute to better blood sugar control and insulin sensitivity.

5. Bone Health:

The alkaline diet's emphasis on alkaline-forming foods can potentially support bone health. Many alkaline foods, such as leafy greens, are rich in calcium, magnesium, and potassium, essential minerals for bone strength. Additionally, the diet avoids acidic foods that may contribute to bone demineralization.

6. Skin Health:

The alkaline lifestyle's focus on consuming antioxidant-rich fruits and vegetables and staying well-hydrated with alkaline water can contribute to healthier skin. Antioxidants help protect the skin from oxidative stress and may promote a more youthful complexion. Proper hydration is also essential for maintaining skin elasticity and preventing dryness.

7. Immune Support:

A well-rounded alkaline diet, packed with vitamins, minerals, and antioxidants, can support a strong immune system. Nutrient-dense foods provide the body with essential nutrients needed to maintain immune function and defend against infections.

8. Athletic Performance:

For athletes, the alkaline lifestyle can provide a good source of energy from nutrient-dense foods. Alkaline-forming foods like fruits and vegetables offer easily digestible carbohydrates and hydration to support endurance and recovery.

9. Cancer Prevention and Recovery:

While the alkaline diet is not a cure for cancer, some studies suggest that consuming a diet rich in fruits and vegetables may be associated with a reduced risk of certain cancers. For individuals undergoing cancer treatment, an alkaline lifestyle can provide valuable nutrients to support overall health and immunity.

10. Hormonal Balance:

The alkaline diet's emphasis on whole, unprocessed foods can support hormonal balance by reducing exposure to hormone-disrupting chemicals found in processed foods. Additionally, maintaining a healthy weight through the alkaline lifestyle can positively impact hormone levels.

11. Alkaline Lifestyle and Detoxification:

The alkaline lifestyle is often associated with detoxification and cleansing the body. Proponents believe that consuming alkaline-forming foods and maintaining a balanced pH can help the body naturally rid itself of toxins and waste products. By prioritizing plant-based, nutrient-dense foods, individuals provide the body with essential nutrients and antioxidants that support the body's detoxification processes.

12. Mental and Emotional Well-being:

The alkaline lifestyle not only focuses on physical health but also emphasizes mental and emotional well-being. Stress-reduction techniques, such as meditation and mindfulness, are often incorporated into the alkaline lifestyle. Additionally, the nutrient-rich diet can positively impact mood and brain health, supporting a more balanced and positive emotional state.

13. Preconception and Pregnancy:

For individuals planning to conceive or during pregnancy, the alkaline lifestyle can provide essential nutrients necessary for reproductive health and fetal development. The diet's emphasis on folate-rich leafy greens and other vitamins and minerals is crucial during this stage. However, pregnant individuals should seek guidance from healthcare professionals to ensure they meet their specific nutritional needs.

14. Anti-Inflammatory Benefits:

The alkaline lifestyle's focus on alkaline-forming foods and avoidance of acidic and inflammatory choices may have potential anti-inflammatory benefits. Chronic inflammation is linked to various health issues, including autoimmune diseases and chronic conditions. Consuming antioxidant-rich fruits and vegetables can help combat inflammation and support overall health.

15. Cancer Recovery Support:

While the alkaline lifestyle is not a standalone treatment for cancer, it can be incorporated as a supportive approach during cancer recovery. Nutrient-dense foods can provide essential vitamins and minerals to strengthen the body during and after cancer treatments. However, it is vital for individuals with cancer to work closely with their healthcare team to develop a comprehensive and evidence-based treatment plan.

16. Age-Related Health Concerns:

As people age, the alkaline lifestyle can play a role in maintaining health and vitality. Consuming a diet rich in alkaline-forming foods, antioxidants, and anti-inflammatory compounds can support aging gracefully and reduce the risk of age-related health issues.

17. Allergies and Sensitivities:

Some individuals with food allergies or sensitivities may find relief in the alkaline lifestyle. By avoiding acidic and potentially triggering foods, individuals can reduce inflammation and digestive distress related to allergens.

18. Gut Health:

The alkaline diet, with its focus on fiber-rich fruits and vegetables, can support gut health by promoting a diverse and healthy gut microbiome. A healthy gut microbiome is essential for digestion, nutrient absorption, and immune function.

Beyond Diet: Embracing a Holistic Alkaline Lifestyle

At the core of Dr. Sebi's teachings was the belief in the power of an alkaline body. While traditional medicine often focuses on treating symptoms, Dr. Sebi's approach was holistic, targeting the root causes of various ailments, which he believed were largely related to the body's pH levels. The fundamental premise is that diseases cannot thrive in an alkaline environment, and thus, by shifting our body's pH to a more alkaline state, we can foster better health and wellness.

But what does it mean to have an "alkaline body"? The pH scale measures how acidic or alkaline a substance is. It ranges from 0 (most acidic) to 14 (most alkaline), with 7 being neutral. Our bodies have a natural pH level of 7.35 to 7.45, which is slightly alkaline. However, many factors, including diet, stress, and environmental toxins, can shift this balance, often making our bodies more acidic.

Beyond Diet: Embracing a Holistic Alkaline Lifestyle

While diet is a critical component in maintaining an alkaline balance, Dr. Sebi believed in a comprehensive approach to health. To truly achieve wellness, one must consider not just what they eat, but also how they live.

1. **Mindfulness and Mental Health**: Stress can lead to acidity in the body. Practices such as meditation, deep breathing exercises, and even simple walks in nature can help reduce stress levels and bring about mental clarity. It's not just about the physical state, but also about achieving mental balance.

2. **Physical Activity**: Regular exercise can help to eliminate acid-forming toxins from the body through sweat. Additionally, certain exercises, especially yoga, focus on deep breathing which can assist in alkalizing the body.

3. **Hydration**: Drinking adequate amounts of water, especially alkaline water, can assist in balancing the body's pH. Water aids in flushing out toxins and acidic waste.

4. **Natural Healing**: Embracing natural remedies and herbs, as suggested by Dr. Sebi, can aid in restoring and maintaining the body's alkaline balance. Plants like burdock root, sarsaparilla, and sea moss were often recommended by him for their healing properties.

5. **Environmental Awareness**: The environment we surround ourselves with plays a pivotal role in our overall well-being. This includes the quality of air we breathe, the products we use, and even the people we surround ourselves with. Opting for natural and organic products, purifying indoor air, and creating a positive and peaceful environment at home can have profound effects on our health.

Book 2: Healing Naturally: Dr. Sebi's Approach to Curing Stds

Understanding Sexually Transmitted Diseases (STDS)

Sexually Transmitted Diseases (STDs), also known as Sexually Transmitted Infections (STIs), are a group of infections that are primarily transmitted through sexual contact. They can affect both men and women of all ages and backgrounds. Understanding STDs is essential for prevention, early detection, and effective treatment. Here are the key aspects of STDs explained in detail:

1. Types of STDs:

There are numerous types of STDs caused by bacteria, viruses, parasites, and fungi. Some common STDs include:

- **Chlamydia:** Caused by the bacterium Chlamydia trachomatis, it often presents with no symptoms but can lead to serious complications if left untreated, such as pelvic inflammatory disease (PID) in women and infertility in both men and women.
- **Gonorrhea:** Caused by the bacterium Neisseria gonorrhoeae, it can cause genital, anal, and throat infections. Like chlamydia, gonorrhea may not always produce noticeable symptoms but can lead to severe health issues if untreated.
- **Human Papillomavirus (HPV):** A viral infection with various strains, some of which can lead to genital warts and an increased risk of cervical, anal, and other types of cancer.
- **Herpes (HSV):** Caused by the herpes simplex virus, there are two types: HSV-1 (typically associated with oral herpes or cold sores) and HSV-2 (commonly associated with genital herpes).
- **Syphilis:** Caused by the bacterium Treponema pallidum, it occurs in stages and can lead to serious complications, including neurological and cardiovascular issues.
- **HIV (Human Immunodeficiency Virus):** A viral infection that attacks the immune system, weakening the body's ability to fight off infections. If left untreated, HIV can progress to AIDS (Acquired Immunodeficiency Syndrome).

2. Modes of Transmission:

STDs are primarily transmitted through sexual contact, including vaginal, anal, and oral sex. They can spread through the exchange of bodily fluids like blood, semen, vaginal fluids, and breast milk. Some STDs, such as HPV and herpes, can also be transmitted through skin-to-skin contact even without penetration.

3. Risk Factors:

Various factors can increase the risk of acquiring an STD, including:

- Having unprotected sex or not using condoms consistently.
- Having multiple sexual partners or engaging in high-risk sexual behaviors.
- A history of prior STD infection.
- Sharing needles or drug equipment for injection drug use.
- Engaging in sexual activities with individuals whose sexual history is unknown or who have a history of STDs.

4. Symptoms:

Symptoms of STDs can vary widely depending on the type of infection, and some infections may not cause any noticeable symptoms at all. Common symptoms may include:

- Genital sores, ulcers, or warts.
- Pain or discomfort during urination or sexual intercourse.
- Abnormal genital discharge.
- Itching, burning, or irritation in the genital area.
- Flu-like symptoms (fever, fatigue) in some cases.

It's crucial to note that many STDs, including chlamydia and gonorrhea, may not cause any symptoms initially, leading to silent infections that can cause complications over time.

5. Complications:

Left untreated, STDs can lead to severe complications, such as:

- Pelvic Inflammatory Disease (PID): A serious infection that can result from untreated chlamydia or gonorrhea, leading to damage to the reproductive organs in women and potentially causing infertility.
- Infertility: Some untreated STDs can lead to scarring and damage to the reproductive organs, affecting fertility in both men and women.
- Increased Risk of HIV Transmission: Some STDs, such as syphilis and genital herpes, can increase the risk of HIV transmission if an individual is exposed to the virus.

- Cervical Cancer: Certain strains of HPV are associated with an increased risk of cervical cancer in women.

6. Prevention and Testing:

Preventing STDs involves practicing safe sex, including consistent and correct condom use, reducing the number of sexual partners, and discussing sexual health with potential partners. Regular testing for STDs is essential, especially for individuals with multiple sexual partners or those engaging in high-risk behaviors. Testing allows for early detection and timely treatment.

7. Treatment and Management:

Many STDs can be treated and managed effectively with appropriate medical care, including antibiotics for bacterial infections and antiviral medications for viral infections like herpes and HIV. Early detection and treatment are crucial to prevent complications and further transmission.

8. Routine Testing and Screenings:

Routine testing and screenings play a significant role in detecting STDs, even in the absence of symptoms. Healthcare providers may recommend regular screenings based on an individual's sexual history, age, and other risk factors. Common tests include:

- **Blood Tests:** Used to detect infections such as HIV, syphilis, and hepatitis B and C.
- **Urine Tests:** Commonly used for diagnosing chlamydia and gonorrhea.
- **Swab Tests:** Used to collect samples from genital, anal, or oral areas to detect infections like HPV, herpes, and bacterial infections.

9. Partner Notification:

If an individual tests positive for an STD, it is essential to inform their sexual partners so they can also get tested and receive appropriate treatment if necessary. Partner notification helps prevent further transmission and allows others to seek timely medical care.

10. Vaccination for Preventable STDs:

Vaccines are available for certain STDs to prevent infection and related complications. For example:

- **HPV Vaccine:** Available for both males and females, it protects against certain strains of

HPV that can lead to genital warts and cervical cancer in women.

- **Hepatitis B Vaccine:** Protects against hepatitis B virus infection, which can be transmitted through sexual contact and other means.
- **HIV Pre-Exposure Prophylaxis (PrEP):** While not a vaccine, PrEP is a preventive medication for individuals at high risk of contracting HIV.

11. Importance of Communication:

Communication is a critical aspect of preventing and managing STDs. Open and honest discussions with sexual partners about sexual history, STD testing, and safe sex practices are essential for reducing the risk of infection.

12. Confidentiality and Non-Judgmental Care:

Healthcare providers play a vital role in ensuring that individuals seeking testing and treatment for STDs feel comfortable and respected. Maintaining confidentiality and providing non-judgmental care create a safe environment for patients to discuss their sexual health openly.

13. The Global Impact of STDs:

STDs are a global public health concern. They affect millions of people worldwide and can have significant social and economic consequences. Various organizations and health initiatives work to raise awareness, provide education, and increase access to testing and treatment to combat the spread of STDs.

14. Stigma and Education:

Stigma surrounding STDs can prevent individuals from seeking testing and treatment. Education and public awareness campaigns aim to reduce stigma, foster empathy, and promote understanding of STDs as common health conditions that can affect anyone.

15. Additional Prevention Measures:

In addition to safe sex practices and vaccination, other prevention measures include:

- **Practicing Abstinence:** Choosing not to engage in sexual activity is a surefire way to prevent STD transmission.
- **Mutual Monogamy:** Being in a sexual relationship with a mutually monogamous

partner who is known to be uninfected reduces the risk of STD transmission.

- **Using Dental Dams and Latex Gloves:** Dental dams and latex gloves can provide protection during oral and manual sex, reducing the risk of STD transmission.

Herbal Remedies for STDS

Herbal remedies have been used for centuries in traditional medicine systems to treat various health conditions, including some symptoms associated with sexually transmitted diseases (STDs). It is crucial to note that while herbal remedies may offer potential benefits, they are not a substitute for medical treatment or professional healthcare advice. If you suspect you have an STD, it is essential to seek medical attention and follow the prescribed treatment plan. Here are some herbal remedies commonly used in traditional medicine for managing certain STD-related symptoms:

1. Echinacea (Echinacea purpurea):

Echinacea is a popular herbal remedy known for its immune-boosting properties. It may be beneficial in supporting the immune system's response to infections, including those associated with STDs. While Echinacea may not directly treat the underlying infection, it could potentially help the body fight off certain pathogens.

2. Garlic (Allium sativum):

Garlic has antimicrobial properties and is believed to have potential benefits in managing certain STDs. It contains allicin, a compound with natural antibiotic properties. Garlic may help combat infections and support overall immune health. However, it is essential to remember that garlic alone is not a replacement for prescribed medical treatment for STDs.

3. Goldenseal (Hydrastis canadensis):

Goldenseal is an herb with natural antimicrobial properties, and it has been traditionally used to address infections, including those affecting the urinary and reproductive systems. However, there is limited scientific evidence to support its effectiveness specifically against STDs. It is essential to use goldenseal with caution and consult with a healthcare professional before using it.

4. Aloe Vera (Aloe barbadensis miller):

Aloe vera has soothing and anti-inflammatory properties, which can be beneficial for managing discomfort and irritation associated with certain STD symptoms, such as genital sores or rashes. Topical application of aloe vera gel may help provide relief, but it will not cure the underlying infection.

5. Licorice (Glycyrrhiza glabra):

Licorice root contains glycyrrhizin, which has antiviral and anti-inflammatory properties. It may potentially offer some benefits in managing herpes and other viral infections associated with STDs. However, it is crucial to use licorice under professional guidance, as excessive consumption can lead to side effects.

6. Neem (Azadirachta indica):

Neem has antimicrobial and antiviral properties, and it has been used traditionally to address various infections. Its potential benefits for managing STD-related symptoms are still being studied, and it is essential to use neem with caution and consult with a healthcare professional.

7. Calendula (Calendula officinalis):

Calendula, also known as marigold, has anti-inflammatory properties and may be used topically to soothe irritated skin and mucous membranes in the genital area. It can be applied as a topical ointment, but it will not treat the underlying infection.

8. Tea Tree Oil (Melaleuca alternifolia):

Tea tree oil has antimicrobial properties and may be used as a topical remedy for certain skin conditions associated with STDs, such as genital warts or herpes sores. However, it is essential to dilute tea tree oil before applying it to the skin and avoid using it internally.

9. Sage (Salvia officinalis):

Sage has antimicrobial and antiviral properties and may offer some benefits for managing infections. It has been traditionally used for various genital and urinary issues. However, its specific effects on STDs are not well-established, and professional guidance is necessary.

10. Cat's Claw (Uncaria tomentosa):

Cat's claw is an herb with immune-modulating properties, and it may support the immune system in managing infections, including those related to STDs. However, more research is needed to establish its efficacy in STD management.

Important Considerations:

- Always consult with a qualified healthcare professional before using herbal remedies, especially if you suspect you have an STD. These remedies should not be used as a replacement for medical treatment or prescribed medications.
- Herbal remedies may interact with medications or other health conditions, so it is crucial to disclose all your health information to your healthcare provider.
- Some herbal remedies may have side effects or adverse reactions, so it is essential to use them with caution and as directed.
- The effectiveness of herbal remedies for managing STDs is still being researched, and more scientific evidence is needed to support their use.

11. Olive Leaf Extract (Olea europaea):

Olive leaf extract is known for its potent antiviral properties. It contains a compound called oleuropein, which has been studied for its ability to combat various viral infections, including those associated with STDs. However, more research is needed to establish its specific efficacy in managing STDs.

12. Astragalus (Astragalus membranaceus):

Astragalus is an herb with immune-boosting properties. It is believed to support the immune system's response to infections, potentially assisting the body in fighting off viral and bacterial pathogens. While it may be used to enhance overall immunity, its direct effects on STDs are not well-documented.

13. Green Tea (Camellia sinensis):

Green tea contains polyphenols, such as catechins, which have antioxidant and antiviral properties. Some studies suggest that green tea may be effective against certain viruses, including herpes simplex virus (HSV). However, further research is needed to determine its efficacy against STDs.

14. St. John's Wort (Hypericum perforatum):

St. John's Wort is an herb with potential antiviral properties. It has been traditionally used to manage viral infections, including herpes. However, its use requires caution, as it can interact with other medications and may have side effects.

15. Propolis:

Propolis is a resin-like substance collected by bees from plants. It contains various compounds with antimicrobial properties, including flavonoids and phenolic acids. Some studies suggest that propolis may have antiviral effects against certain pathogens, but more research is needed to understand its specific role in managing STDs.

16. Pau d'Arco (Tabebuia avellanedae):

Pau d'Arco is an herb traditionally used for its antifungal and antimicrobial properties. It may have potential benefits for managing certain infections associated with STDs. However, its use should be supervised by a healthcare professional.

17. Burdock Root (Arctium lappa):

Burdock root is known for its cleansing and detoxifying properties. It may support the body's natural detoxification processes, potentially aiding in the elimination of waste and toxins associated with certain infections. However, its direct effects on STDs are not well-established.

18. Turmeric (Curcuma longa):

Turmeric contains a compound called curcumin, which has potent anti-inflammatory and antioxidant properties. It may be used to support the body's immune response and reduce inflammation associated with certain STD symptoms. However, it is essential to use turmeric as a complementary approach and not as a replacement for medical treatment.

Alkaline Diet and STDS

Dr. Sebi's approach to healing was deeply rooted in the power of nature. He believed that the body has the intrinsic ability to heal itself, provided it is given the right conditions. One of the more controversial claims he made during his life was that he had found natural remedies capable of curing a number of sexually transmitted infections (STIs).

According to Dr. Sebi, most diseases, including STIs, thrive in an acidic environment. By creating a more alkaline environment within the body, he postulated that these diseases could be naturally suppressed or even eliminated. His approach combined natural herbs with a strict diet, emphasizing the consumption of what he labeled "electric foods." These foods are believed to nourish the body at the cellular level, promoting healing and reducing the body's mucus buildup, which he believed was a primary source of disease.

Alkaline Diet and STIs

The alkaline diet recommended by Dr. Sebi is a plant-based diet that avoids processed foods, sugars, dairy, and meats. The main focus is on raw fruits, vegetables, nuts, seeds, and grains that are alkaline-forming. Here's how this approach could potentially relate to STIs:

1. **Natural Immunity Boost**: An alkaline diet rich in vitamins, minerals, and antioxidants is believed to strengthen the immune system. A robust immune system is crucial in battling infections, including STIs.

2. **Reduced Inflammation**: Foods high in alkalinity are anti-inflammatory by nature. Inflammation is often associated with disease progression. By reducing inflammation, the body may be better equipped to heal.

3. **Herbal Remedies**: Along with an alkaline diet, Dr. Sebi recommended specific herbs that are believed to have potent healing properties. For instance, herbs like cascara sagrada and chaparral were touted for their cleansing and anti-viral properties, respectively.

4. **Detoxification**: The combination of an alkaline diet and specific herbs can support the body's natural detoxification process. By eliminating toxins and mucus buildup, the body may have a better environment to combat infections.

The Power of Nature in Healing

Dr. Sebi's philosophy wasn't just about countering diseases but about achieving a state of holistic wellness where the body operates at its optimal level. Central to his teachings was the understanding that nature, in its original form, provides all the tools necessary for the human body to thrive.

1. **Bio-mineral Balance**: Dr. Sebi emphasized the importance of the body's bio-mineral balance. He believed that many of the common ailments people suffer from are due to the body being out of balance, mainly due to a lack of essential minerals. By restoring this balance through foods and herbs that are naturally rich in these minerals, he believed the body could rejuvenate and heal itself.

2. **Electric Foods**: These are foods that are not hybrids and have not been modified from their original state. According to Dr. Sebi, electric foods resonate with the electric body, nourishing and revitalizing it in a way that hybrid or modified foods can't. Examples include wild berries, walnuts, and certain grains like quinoa and kamut.

3. **Mucus-reducing Foods**: A significant pillar of Dr. Sebi's teachings revolved around the concept that mucus buildup in the body was a significant contributor to disease. He contended that diseases would manifest in areas where mucus accumulation was highest. To combat this, he recommended a diet that was devoid of mucus-forming foods like dairy and meat, focusing instead on foods that naturally reduce mucus production.

4. **The Power of Fasting**: Dr. Sebi was also a proponent of periodic fasting, believing that giving the digestive system a break allowed the body to focus on healing and detoxification. Combined with his recommended herbal treatments, fasting was viewed as a potent tool to reset and rejuvenate the body.

5. **Community and Support**: Beyond just the physical aspects of health, Dr. Sebi recognized the importance of a supportive community. Being surrounded by like-minded individuals who encourage and uphold these natural principles can make the journey toward health more manageable and sustainable.

Holistic Approaches to Long-Term Healing

Holistic Sexually transmitted infections (STIs) are conventionally treated with medications, typically antibiotics or antivirals, depending on the nature of the infection. Dr. Sebi, however, viewed STIs, like all diseases, through a holistic lens. Here's how he approached the long-term healing of STIs using a comprehensive methodology:

1. **Dietary Emphasis**: Dr. Sebi often highlighted that mucus buildup in the body was a significant contributor to disease, including STIs. He proposed a diet rich in alkaline foods, which naturally reduce mucus production. By consuming foods like kale, mushrooms, quinoa, and rye, one could potentially create an environment less conducive to the thriving of infections.

2. **Detoxification**: To combat STIs, Dr. Sebi emphasized the importance of detoxifying the body. This would involve not only consuming alkaline foods but also integrating specific herbs into one's regimen. These herbs would assist in purging the body of toxins and excess mucus, which he believed to be linked to disease progression.

3. **Stress Management**: Stress, both physical and emotional, can weaken the immune system, making the body more susceptible to infections and reducing its ability to fight existing ones. Mindfulness practices, meditation, and connecting with nature were among Dr. Sebi's recommended tools to manage and reduce stress.

4. **Herbal Protocols**: Dr. Sebi suggested a range of herbs, believed to possess antiviral and antibacterial properties, for combating STIs. Some herbs like sarsaparilla were known for their immune-boosting properties, while others like cascara sagrada aided in detoxification.

5. **Immunity Enhancement**: To holistically approach STIs, one must focus on fortifying the body's natural defenses. Foods rich in vitamins and minerals, like seamoss and bladderwrack, were considered pivotal in this approach. Coupled with herbs and an alkaline diet, the aim was to create a fortified body less prone to infections and more capable of healing.

6. **Emotional and Spiritual Health**: Emotional traumas and suppressed emotions can

manifest as physical ailments. Dr. Sebi believed that true healing, especially for long-term issues like STIs, required addressing emotional and spiritual well-being. Practices that nurture the spirit, provide emotional release, and promote mental clarity were integral to his holistic approach to STIs.

Book 3: Herpes No More: Dr. Sebi's Natural Remedies for Herpes

Understanding Herpes: Types and Symptoms

Herpes is a common viral infection caused by the herpes simplex virus (HSV). There are two main types of herpes viruses: herpes simplex virus type 1 (HSV-1) and herpes simplex virus type 2 (HSV-2). Understanding the types and symptoms of herpes is essential for recognizing and managing this widespread infection.

Herpes Simplex Virus Type 1 (HSV-1):

Transmission: HSV-1 is typically associated with oral herpes and is often transmitted through oral-to-oral contact. It can also be spread through sharing utensils, towels, or through close contact with an infected individual's saliva.

Symptoms: HSV-1 commonly causes oral herpes, which is characterized by cold sores or fever blisters around the mouth or on the lips. These sores are often painful, itchy, and can be accompanied by tingling or burning sensations before they appear. Cold sores can last for about a week and may recur periodically, especially during times of stress or illness.

Herpes Simplex Virus Type 2 (HSV-2):

Transmission: HSV-2 is primarily associated with genital herpes and is typically transmitted through sexual contact, including vaginal, anal, and oral sex. It can also be spread from a pregnant person to their newborn during childbirth.

Symptoms: Genital herpes caused by HSV-2 leads to the formation of painful, fluid-filled blisters or ulcers in the genital and anal areas. These blisters can cause discomfort, itching, and pain during urination. Like oral herpes, genital herpes symptoms can come and go, with recurrent outbreaks triggered by factors such as stress, illness, or hormonal changes.

Commonalities and Differences:

While HSV-1 is traditionally linked to oral herpes and HSV-2 to genital herpes, both types can cause infections in either location. This is due to the increasing prevalence of oral-genital contact, which has led to HSV-1 causing genital herpes and HSV-2 causing oral herpes in some cases.

Asymptomatic Carriers:

It's important to note that many people infected with HSV-1 or HSV-2 may not experience noticeable symptoms. These individuals are considered asymptomatic carriers, and they can still transmit the virus to others through viral shedding, even if they don't have active sores.

Diagnosis:

Diagnosing herpes involves clinical evaluation, physical examination, and sometimes laboratory tests. Doctors may perform viral culture tests, polymerase chain reaction (PCR) tests, or antibody blood tests to confirm the presence of the virus.

Prevention and Management:

- **Safe Sex Practices:** Consistent and correct use of condoms or dental dams during sexual activity can reduce the risk of transmitting and contracting genital herpes.
- **Antiviral Medications:** Antiviral drugs can help manage herpes symptoms and reduce the frequency and severity of outbreaks. They may also reduce the risk of transmitting the virus to sexual partners.
- **Communication:** Openly discussing your herpes status with sexual partners is crucial for informed decision-making and reducing the risk of transmission.
- **Stress Management:** Stress can trigger herpes outbreaks. Practicing stress reduction techniques such as meditation, yoga, and exercise can help manage symptoms.
- **Avoiding Triggers:** Identifying and avoiding triggers that may induce outbreaks, such as certain foods or emotional stress, can help manage herpes symptoms.

Herpes Transmission and Stigma:

It's important to address the stigma surrounding herpes. Due to the cultural and social perceptions of the virus, individuals diagnosed with herpes may face emotional challenges, feelings of shame, and fear of judgment. Education and open conversations about herpes can help reduce stigma, foster empathy, and create a more supportive environment for those living with the infection.

Complications and Risks:

While herpes outbreaks are often manageable, there are certain considerations to be aware of:

- **Pregnancy:** Pregnant individuals with genital herpes should inform their healthcare provider. There is a risk of transmitting the virus to the newborn during childbirth, which can lead to severe complications.
- **HIV Risk:** Herpes infection can increase the risk of contracting or transmitting the human immunodeficiency virus (HIV) during sexual contact, as open sores provide entry points for the virus.
- **Rare Complications:** In rare cases, the herpes virus can cause more severe complications, such as herpes encephalitis (inflammation of the brain) or ocular herpes (infection of the eye). These complications require immediate medical attention.

Support and Resources:

For individuals diagnosed with herpes, seeking support and accurate information is essential. There are numerous resources available, including:

- **Healthcare Providers:** Consult with healthcare professionals for accurate diagnosis, treatment options, and guidance on managing herpes.
- **Sexual Health Clinics:** Sexual health clinics offer testing, counseling, and support for individuals with herpes.
- **Online Communities:** Online support groups and forums allow individuals to connect with others who have herpes, share experiences, and receive emotional support.
- **Educational Websites:** Reputable websites from health organizations provide accurate information about herpes, its symptoms, transmission, and management.

Dr. Sebi's Herbal Recommendations for Herpes

Dr. Sebi, whose full name is Alfredo Darrington Bowman, was a self-proclaimed herbalist and natural healer known for his unique dietary and herbal recommendations. He believed in the concept of maintaining an alkaline body pH to support overall health and well-being. While Dr. Sebi's approach to health has garnered attention and followers, it's important to note that his methods are not supported by mainstream medical research and have been met with skepticism by medical professionals.

Dr. Sebi's Approach to Herpes:

Dr. Sebi's approach to managing herpes focused on alkaline foods and herbal remedies to create an environment in the body that he believed would discourage the growth of viruses, including herpes. He emphasized the consumption of plant-based, whole foods and herbal formulations to support the body's natural healing processes.

Herbs and Herbal Recommendations:

Dr. Sebi recommended several herbs and herbal compounds that he believed could be beneficial for managing herpes symptoms. Some of these herbs include:

- **Bladderwrack:** A type of seaweed rich in minerals, including iodine, which Dr. Sebi believed could help balance the body's pH and support the immune system.
- **Burdock Root:** Known for its potential anti-inflammatory and detoxifying properties, burdock root was suggested by Dr. Sebi to support overall health and immune function.
- **Echinacea:** Dr. Sebi believed that echinacea could strengthen the immune system and assist the body in fighting infections, including herpes.
- **Irish Moss:** A type of seaweed rich in nutrients, Irish moss was recommended by Dr. Sebi for its potential to support the body's alkalinity and overall health.
- **Dandelion:** Dr. Sebi suggested that dandelion could support detoxification processes in the body and promote optimal functioning.
- **Aloe Vera:** Known for its soothing and anti-inflammatory properties, aloe vera was recommended by Dr. Sebi as part of an alkaline diet.

Important Considerations:

- Dr. Sebi's recommendations are not backed by scientific evidence and are not endorsed by mainstream medical organizations. His approach has been criticized for lacking rigorous scientific research to support its claims.
- The effectiveness of the herbs and remedies suggested by Dr. Sebi for managing herpes has not been verified through clinical trials or scientific studies.
- Herpes is a complex viral infection, and managing it requires medical guidance, antiviral medications (if recommended by healthcare professionals), and safe sex practices.
- If you are considering using herbs or supplements, consult with a healthcare provider before doing so. Some herbs may interact with medications or have contraindications, especially if you have underlying health conditions.
- Dr. Sebi's dietary recommendations may involve avoiding certain foods that are commonly included in a balanced diet, and this could potentially impact nutritional intake.

Scientific Perspective and Clinical Evidence:

- It's important to highlight that Dr. Sebi's herbal recommendations lack the rigorous scientific validation typically required in mainstream medicine. While certain herbs he suggested may have potential health benefits, their effectiveness in treating or managing herpes has not been substantiated through clinical trials or well-established research. The scientific community generally relies on evidence-based medicine, where treatments and interventions are thoroughly tested and proven before being recommended.

Alkaline Diet and Overall Health:

- Dr. Sebi's emphasis on consuming alkaline foods is based on the belief that an alkaline body pH can create an environment less conducive to viral growth. However, the human body naturally regulates its pH, and the impact of dietary pH on herpes or other viral infections is not well-supported by scientific evidence. While adopting a diet rich in fruits, vegetables, and whole foods is generally beneficial for overall health, its direct impact on managing herpes is not definitively established.

Collaboration with Healthcare Professionals:

- Individuals considering Dr. Sebi's herbal recommendations should consult with a qualified healthcare provider before making any significant changes to their diet or incorporating herbal supplements. Healthcare professionals can offer personalized guidance, assess potential interactions with medications, and provide a balanced perspective on alternative approaches.

Medical Treatment and Preventive Measures:

- While Dr. Sebi's herbal recommendations may hold appeal for some individuals seeking natural remedies, it's important to remember that medical treatment remains a cornerstone of managing herpes. Antiviral medications prescribed by healthcare providers can help manage symptoms, reduce the frequency and severity of outbreaks, and lower the risk of transmitting the virus to sexual partners.

Safe Sex Practices and Communication:

- Regardless of any alternative approaches considered, practicing safe sex and open communication with sexual partners about herpes status are crucial for preventing transmission. Condom use, dental dams, and regular testing are vital components of preventing the spread of herpes and other sexually transmitted infections.

Adopting an Alkaline Diet for Herpes Management

An alkaline diet is based on the concept that consuming foods that promote an alkaline pH in the body can support overall health and potentially impact the management of health conditions, including herpes. While there is limited scientific evidence directly linking the alkaline diet to herpes management, adopting a diet rich in nutrient-dense, alkaline-forming foods can have potential benefits for overall well-being. Here's a detailed explanation of how to adopt an alkaline diet for herpes management:

1. Understanding pH Balance:

The body's pH level refers to its acidity or alkalinity. Proponents of the alkaline diet believe that maintaining a slightly alkaline pH can create an environment less conducive to viral replication and inflammation. However, the human body's pH is naturally regulated, and dietary factors have a limited impact on this balance.

2. Focus on Alkaline-Forming Foods:

An alkaline diet emphasizes foods that have an alkalizing effect on the body, such as fruits, vegetables, nuts, seeds, and legumes. These foods are typically nutrient-dense, rich in vitamins, minerals, antioxidants, and fiber.

3. Emphasize Plant-Based Foods:

The foundation of an alkaline diet is plant-based foods. Aim to fill your plate with a variety of colorful fruits and vegetables, as they are naturally alkaline-forming and provide essential nutrients that support immune function and overall health.

4. Include Leafy Greens:

Leafy greens like kale, spinach, and Swiss chard are excellent choices for an alkaline diet. They are rich in chlorophyll and minerals that can help maintain a balanced pH.

5. Opt for Whole Grains:

Choose whole grains such as quinoa, brown rice, and oats over refined grains. Whole grains provide complex carbohydrates, fiber, and important nutrients that contribute to overall well-being.

6. Incorporate Healthy Fats:

Include sources of healthy fats like avocados, nuts, seeds, and olive oil. These fats support cardiovascular health and provide satiety.

7. Limit Acid-Forming Foods:

While an alkaline diet encourages alkaline-forming foods, it also suggests limiting acid-forming foods, such as processed foods, sugar, refined grains, and excessive animal products. These foods are believed to contribute to an acidic environment in the body.

8. Stay Hydrated:

Drinking plenty of water is essential for maintaining overall health and supporting bodily functions. Aim to stay well-hydrated throughout the day.

9. Alkaline Beverages:

Incorporate alkaline beverages like herbal teas, green juices, and smoothies made with alkaline-forming ingredients. These can contribute to your hydration while also providing valuable nutrients.

10. Moderate Protein Intake:

Include plant-based protein sources like beans, lentils, tofu, and tempeh. These options are less acidic than animal-based proteins and provide essential amino acids.

11. Portion Control:

Practice portion control to prevent overeating, as excessive consumption of even alkaline foods can lead to weight gain and potential health imbalances.

12. Mindful Eating:

Practice mindful eating by paying attention to hunger and fullness cues. Chew food thoroughly and savor the flavors, which can promote digestion and nutrient absorption.

13. Variety and Balance:

Maintaining variety in your alkaline diet is important to ensure you receive a wide range of nutrients. Rotate your food choices to include different fruits, vegetables, grains, and legumes. This diversity helps provide essential vitamins, minerals, and antioxidants that contribute to your overall health.

14. Mindful Carbohydrate Choices:

Carbohydrates are a significant part of the alkaline diet. Opt for complex carbohydrates found in whole grains, vegetables, and fruits, which provide sustained energy and fiber, promoting digestion and satiety.

15. Alkaline Snacking:

Choose alkaline snacks such as raw vegetables with hummus, mixed nuts, seeds, and fresh fruit. These options can help maintain your alkaline balance and provide nourishment between meals.

16. Portion of Animal-Based Foods:

If you choose to include animal-based foods in your diet, do so in moderation. Lean toward lean poultry, fish, and eggs. These choices are considered less acidic than red meats.

17. Monitoring Personal Response:

As with any dietary approach, pay attention to how your body responds to changes. Some individuals may experience improved energy levels, digestion, or overall well-being when adopting an alkaline diet, while others may not notice significant changes.

18. Whole Foods Approach:

The alkaline diet encourages a whole foods approach by minimizing processed and refined foods. Processed foods often contain additives, preservatives, and excess sodium, which can contribute to an acidic environment in the body.

19. Consulting a Healthcare Professional:

Before making significant dietary changes, especially if you're managing a health condition like herpes, consult with a healthcare provider. They can offer personalized guidance, ensure that your nutritional needs are met, and advise you on how dietary changes may interact with your medical treatment.

20. Emotional Well-Being:

Remember that overall well-being extends beyond diet. Managing herpes also involves stress reduction, emotional support, and open communication with sexual partners and healthcare professionals.

21. Safe Sex Practices:

While diet can play a role in supporting overall health, preventing transmission of herpes through safe sex practices is equally important. Use condoms or dental dams correctly and consistently during sexual activity to reduce the risk of spreading the virus.

Book 4: HIV-Free Living: Dr. Sebi's Holistic Solutions for HIV

Understanding HIV: Transmission and Progression

HIV (Human Immunodeficiency Virus) is a virus that attacks the immune system, weakening the body's ability to fight off infections and diseases. Understanding how HIV is transmitted and how it progresses is crucial for preventing its spread and managing its impact on health. Let's delve into the details:

1. Transmission of HIV:

- **Explanation:** HIV is primarily transmitted through certain body fluids, including blood, semen, vaginal fluids, rectal fluids, and breast milk. The most common modes of transmission include:
  - Unprotected sexual intercourse: HIV can be transmitted through vaginal, anal, or oral sex with an infected partner, especially if there are open sores, cuts, or mucous membranes involved.
  - Sharing needles: Injecting drugs using contaminated needles or syringes can transmit HIV.
  - Mother-to-child transmission: HIV can be transmitted from an infected mother to her baby during pregnancy, childbirth, or breastfeeding.
  - Blood transfusions: Though rare now due to stringent screening, blood transfusions with contaminated blood can transmit HIV.

2. Progression of HIV:

- **Explanation:** After infection with HIV, there are several stages of disease progression:
  - Acute HIV infection: This initial phase occurs within 2 to 4 weeks after exposure. Some people experience flu-like symptoms, while others may not have noticeable symptoms.
  - Clinical latency (chronic) stage: After the acute phase, HIV enters a dormant period where the virus reproduces at low levels. This stage can last for years with few or no symptoms.
  - AIDS (Acquired Immunodeficiency Syndrome): If HIV is left untreated, it can lead to AIDS, the final stage of HIV infection. AIDS is characterized by a severely compromised

immune system, making the body susceptible to opportunistic infections and certain cancers.

3. Impact on Immune System:

- **Explanation:** HIV attacks CD4 T cells, a type of white blood cell crucial for maintaining a healthy immune system. As the virus replicates and destroys these cells, the immune system becomes weakened, increasing vulnerability to infections and diseases.

4. Management and Treatment:

- **Explanation:** Antiretroviral therapy (ART) is the standard treatment for HIV. ART helps control the virus, prevent or slow the progression of HIV, and reduce the risk of transmission. When taken consistently and as prescribed, ART can allow individuals with HIV to live long and healthy lives.

5. Prevention:

- **Explanation:** Preventing the transmission of HIV involves several strategies:
  - Practicing safe sex: Using condoms consistently and correctly during sexual activity can greatly reduce the risk of HIV transmission.
  - Getting tested and knowing your partner's status: Regular HIV testing and open communication with sexual partners can help prevent the spread of HIV.
  - Using clean needles: If injecting drugs, using clean needles and not sharing injecting equipment can prevent HIV transmission.
  - Preventing mother-to-child transmission: Pregnant women with HIV can take medication to prevent transmitting the virus to their babies.

Conclusion:

Understanding the transmission and progression of HIV is essential for promoting awareness, prevention, and proper management. Timely testing, access to treatment, and adopting safe behaviors contribute to reducing the spread of HIV and improving the quality of life for those living with the virus. If you have concerns about HIV, it's advisable to consult with healthcare professionals who specialize in HIV care and prevention.

Dr. Sebi's Herbal Support for HIV

Dr. Sebi's approach to health and well-being involves utilizing natural herbs and plant-based foods to support the body's natural healing processes. While there is no known cure for HIV, some individuals may seek herbal and nutritional support to complement their medical treatment. Here's an in-depth explanation of some of the herbs Dr. Sebi recommended for supporting overall health and immune function in the context of HIV:

1. Burdock Root:

- **Explanation:** Burdock root is known for its potential immune-boosting properties. It may help support detoxification, improve digestion, and promote healthy skin. Some herbalists suggest it could be beneficial for individuals with chronic infections.

2. Irish Sea Moss:

- **Explanation:** Irish sea moss is rich in minerals and nutrients that support immune function and overall health. It contains vitamins, minerals, and trace elements that can aid in maintaining the body's vitality.

3. Bladderwrack:

- **Explanation:** Bladderwrack is another seaweed that Dr. Sebi recommended. It's believed to be a source of essential minerals that support thyroid health and overall well-being.

4. Elderberry:

- **Explanation:** Elderberry is known for its potential immune-strengthening properties. It's rich in antioxidants and vitamins that can help the body fight off infections and maintain overall health.

5. Chaparral:

- **Explanation:** Chaparral is an herb that has been used traditionally for its potential immune-boosting and detoxifying properties. It's important to note that there have been concerns about potential toxicity, so its use should be approached cautiously and under the guidance of a healthcare professional.

6. Dandelion:

- **Explanation:** Dandelion is believed to support detoxification and liver health. A healthy liver is crucial for overall immune function and maintaining vitality.

7. Sarsaparilla:

- **Explanation:** Sarsaparilla has been used traditionally for its potential anti-inflammatory and immune-modulating properties. It may help the body manage inflammation and support immune response.

8. Yellow Dock:

- **Explanation:** Yellow dock is believed to support detoxification and digestive health. A healthy digestive system is essential for proper nutrient absorption and overall well-being.

Note: It's important to emphasize that while these herbs have been traditionally used for various health benefits, there is limited scientific evidence to support their specific effects on HIV. People living with HIV should consult with a healthcare professional before incorporating any herbs into their treatment plan, as herbs can interact with medications and may have different effects on each individual.

The Alkaline Diet for HIV Management

In the sphere of holistic wellness, Dr. Sebi's teachings emphasized the significance of the body's internal environment. His perspective on managing conditions like HIV was centered around the belief that a body in harmony, especially at a cellular level, could be more resilient and better equipped to face health challenges.

The alkaline diet, as championed by Dr. Sebi, is based on the idea that certain foods can influence the body's pH levels. While the human body has various pH levels depending on the organ or system, Sebi's dietary guidelines aimed to create a more alkaline environment in the body, reducing the overall acidity. It was his assertion that a less acidic environment could potentially make it harder for diseases to thrive.

Detoxification is another aspect that was integral to Dr. Sebi's approach. He believed that by ridding the body of toxins and impurities, one could pave the way for better absorption of essential nutrients. For an individual managing HIV, a system that efficiently absorbs nutrients can be critical in maintaining health and vitality. By introducing foods that are naturally detoxifying, such as leafy greens, fresh fruits, and non-hybrid grains, Sebi believed one could cleanse the system and rejuvenate the cells.

Furthermore, the emphasis on avoiding mucus-forming foods stems from Dr. Sebi's theory linking mucus buildup to disease proliferation. For him, foods like dairy, certain meats, and processed foods could lead to excessive mucus, potentially obstructing the body's natural functions. By eliminating these foods, he believed one could clear pathways, thus enhancing the body's natural healing capabilities.

Herbal remedies have always been a pillar of Dr. Sebi's approach to wellness. He often spoke about the therapeutic benefits of herbs, not just for their nutrient content but also for their potential to support the body's healing processes. Plants like elderberry, which is often hailed for its immune-boosting properties, or burdock root, known for its blood purifying qualities, were regularly recommended in his protocols.

Lastly, the mental and emotional well-being of an individual was an aspect Dr. Sebi never overlooked. He frequently underlined the connection between the mind and body, asserting that emotional traumas and unresolved stress could manifest as physical ailments. By fostering practices that encourage mental clarity, stress relief, and emotional release, he believed one could achieve a state of balance, vital for long-term wellness.

Embracing Positivity and Hope: Living Fully with HIV

Living with HIV presents challenges, but it's also an opportunity to cultivate a positive mindset, focus on hope, and embrace life to the fullest. With the right strategies and perspectives, individuals with HIV can lead fulfilling and joyful lives. Here's an in-depth exploration of how to embrace positivity and hope while living with HIV:

1. Self-Empowerment:

- **Explanation:** Empowerment comes from understanding that you have the ability to take control of your life and make choices that positively impact your well-being. Educate yourself about HIV, treatment options, and ways to support your health.

2. Gratitude and Mindfulness:

- **Explanation:** Practicing gratitude and mindfulness can shift your focus from challenges to the present moment. Mindfulness techniques, such as meditation and deep breathing, can reduce stress and foster a positive mindset.

3. Setting Goals:

- **Explanation:** Setting achievable goals—whether they're related to health, personal growth, career, or relationships—can provide a sense of purpose and direction. Celebrating small victories along the way boosts self-esteem.

4. Support Systems:

- **Explanation:** Surround yourself with a supportive network of friends, family, healthcare professionals, and support groups. Having people who understand, listen, and encourage you contributes to a positive outlook.

5. Resilience Building:

- **Explanation:** Cultivate resilience by viewing challenges as opportunities for growth. Resilience allows you to bounce back from setbacks and keep moving forward.

6. Sharing Your Story:

- **Explanation:** Sharing your journey and experiences with others can foster connection, break down stigma, and inspire hope. Your story has the power to uplift and educate others.

7. Pursuing Passions:

- **Explanation:** Engage in activities that bring you joy and fulfillment. Pursuing hobbies, creative endeavors, or activities you're passionate about can boost mood and overall well-being.

8. Celebrating Life:

- **Explanation:** Celebrate milestones and special moments in your life. Recognizing achievements, both big and small, reinforces the positivity in your journey.

9. Continued Learning:

- **Explanation:** Stay informed about advancements in HIV research, treatment options, and self-care strategies. Knowledge empowers you to make informed decisions and take control of your health.

10. Supporting Others:

- **Explanation:** Being a source of support for others living with HIV or those who may be at risk can provide a sense of purpose and satisfaction. Offering guidance and understanding fosters a sense of community.

Book 5: Defeating Diabetes: Dr. Sebi's Path to Reversing Diabetes Naturally

Understanding Diabetes: Types and Risk Factors

Diabetes is a chronic metabolic disorder characterized by high blood sugar levels (hyperglycemia) due to either insufficient insulin production or poor utilization of insulin by the body. Insulin is a hormone produced by the pancreas that regulates blood sugar. There are different types of diabetes, each with its own causes, characteristics, and risk factors. Let's delve into the details of diabetes types and associated risk factors:

Types of Diabetes:

1. **Type 1 Diabetes:** Type 1 diabetes, often referred to as juvenile diabetes, is an autoimmune condition where the immune system mistakenly attacks and destroys the insulin-producing cells in the pancreas. This results in little to no insulin production. Individuals with type 1 diabetes require insulin injections or insulin pumps to manage their blood sugar levels.

2. **Type 2 Diabetes:** Type 2 diabetes is the most common form of diabetes. It occurs when the body becomes resistant to insulin or doesn't produce enough insulin to maintain normal blood sugar levels. This type is often associated with lifestyle factors such as obesity, physical inactivity, and poor dietary choices.

3. **Gestational Diabetes:** Gestational diabetes occurs during pregnancy when hormonal changes lead to insulin resistance. It usually resolves after childbirth, but it increases the risk of both the mother and child developing type 2 diabetes later in life.

4. **Other Specific Types:** There are other rare forms of diabetes caused by specific genetic mutations, diseases, medications, or pancreatic conditions.

Risk Factors for Type 2 Diabetes:

1. **Obesity:** Excess body weight, particularly around the abdomen, increases the risk of type 2 diabetes. Obesity contributes to insulin resistance and inflammation.

2. **Physical Inactivity:** A sedentary lifestyle reduces the body's ability to effectively use insulin and control blood sugar levels.

3. **Unhealthy Diet:** Diets high in refined sugars, saturated and trans fats, and low in fiber contribute to the development of type 2 diabetes. Poor nutrition affects insulin

sensitivity and metabolism.

4. **Family History:** Having a family history of diabetes increases the risk, suggesting a genetic predisposition.

5. **Age:** The risk of type 2 diabetes increases with age, particularly after 45 years. This is partly due to reduced physical activity and muscle mass.

6. **Ethnicity:** Some ethnic groups, such as African-Americans, Hispanics, Native Americans, and Asians, have a higher risk of developing diabetes.

7. **Gestational Diabetes:** Women who have had gestational diabetes or have given birth to large babies are at a higher risk of developing type 2 diabetes.

8. **Polycystic Ovary Syndrome (PCOS):** Women with PCOS, a hormonal disorder, are at an increased risk of developing insulin resistance and type 2 diabetes.

9. **Hypertension (High Blood Pressure):** High blood pressure is linked to an increased risk of developing type 2 diabetes.

10. **High Cholesterol Levels:** Abnormal lipid levels, including high triglycerides and low HDL ("good") cholesterol, can increase the risk of diabetes.

Types of Diabetes:

1. **Type 1 Diabetes:** Type 1 diabetes, often diagnosed in childhood or adolescence, results from the immune system attacking and destroying the insulin-producing cells (beta cells) in the pancreas. This leads to an absolute lack of insulin production. People with type 1 diabetes require insulin injections or infusion through an insulin pump to manage their blood sugar levels.

2. **Type 2 Diabetes:** Type 2 diabetes is characterized by insulin resistance, where the body's cells do not respond effectively to insulin. As a result, blood sugar levels rise. Initially, the pancreas produces more insulin to compensate, but over time, it may not keep up with the demand. This form of diabetes is closely linked to lifestyle factors such as obesity, physical inactivity, and poor dietary habits.

3. **Gestational Diabetes:** Gestational diabetes occurs during pregnancy when hormonal changes and insulin resistance lead to elevated blood sugar levels. While it usually resolves after childbirth, women who have had gestational diabetes have an increased risk of developing type 2 diabetes later in life.

4. **Other Specific Types:** There are rarer forms of diabetes caused by specific factors, such as genetic mutations, diseases of the pancreas, certain medications, and endocrine disorders.

Risk Factors for Type 2 Diabetes:

1. **Obesity:** Excess body weight, particularly abdominal obesity, is a major risk factor for type 2 diabetes. Fat cells release chemicals that contribute to insulin resistance.

2. **Physical Inactivity:** Lack of regular physical activity reduces the body's ability to use insulin effectively and control blood sugar levels.

3. **Unhealthy Diet:** Diets high in sugary beverages, processed foods, and unhealthy fats contribute to obesity and insulin resistance.

4. **Family History:** Having a close family member with diabetes increases the risk, suggesting a genetic predisposition.

5. **Age:** The risk of type 2 diabetes increases with age, especially after 45. This may be due to factors like decreased physical activity and muscle mass.

6. **Ethnicity:** Certain ethnic groups, including African-Americans, Hispanics, Native Americans, and Asians, have a higher risk of developing type 2 diabetes.

7. **Gestational Diabetes:** Women who have had gestational diabetes during pregnancy are at a higher risk of developing type 2 diabetes.

8. **Polycystic Ovary Syndrome (PCOS):** Women with PCOS, a hormonal disorder, are at an increased risk of insulin resistance and type 2 diabetes.

9. **Hypertension (High Blood Pressure):** High blood pressure is linked to an increased risk of type 2 diabetes.

10. **High Cholesterol Levels:** Abnormal lipid levels, including high triglycerides and low HDL ("good") cholesterol, can increase the risk of diabetes.

Dr. Sebi's Herbal Remedies for Diabetes

Dr. Sebi, also known as Alfredo Darrington Bowman, was a Honduran herbalist and self-proclaimed healer who gained popularity for his alternative approach to health and wellness. He advocated for a plant-based, alkaline diet and promoted various herbal remedies for various health conditions, including diabetes. However, it's important to note that Dr. Sebi's claims and recommendations lack scientific validation and are not endorsed by mainstream medical authorities. Let's explore some of the herbal remedies he suggested for diabetes:

1. Sea Moss (Irish Moss):

Dr. Sebi often mentioned sea moss as a nutrient-rich seaweed that he believed could help regulate blood sugar levels. Sea moss is a source of vitamins, minerals, and dietary fiber, which can have overall health benefits. However, there is limited scientific evidence directly linking sea moss consumption to diabetes management.

2. Blue Vervain:

Dr. Sebi recommended blue vervain as an herbal remedy for diabetes. Blue vervain is traditionally used for various purposes, including relaxation and calming effects. However, its effectiveness in managing diabetes has not been scientifically proven.

3. Sage:

Sage is another herb Dr. Sebi suggested for diabetes. Some research suggests that sage may have potential benefits for blood sugar regulation, but more studies are needed to establish its effectiveness as a diabetes treatment.

4. Burdock Root:

Dr. Sebi mentioned burdock root as an herb that could potentially help with diabetes. Burdock root is known for its potential diuretic and antioxidant properties, but its specific impact on diabetes management requires further investigation.

5. Herbal Teas:

Dr. Sebi often recommended herbal teas made from various plants as part of his approach. Some of these teas, such as chamomile and ginger, have potential health benefits, but their direct impact on diabetes management is not well-established.

6. Bitter Melon:

Bitter melon is a plant often suggested as a natural remedy for diabetes in traditional medicine practices. Some studies have shown that bitter melon may have blood sugar-lowering effects, but more research is needed to determine its efficacy and safety for diabetes management.

7. Aloe Vera:

Aloe vera is known for its soothing properties and is sometimes recommended by alternative practitioners for diabetes. Some research suggests that aloe vera may have a modest impact on reducing blood sugar levels, but its long-term safety and effectiveness are still under investigation.

8. Nopal (Prickly Pear Cactus):

Dr. Sebi also mentioned nopal as a potential remedy for diabetes. Nopal is rich in fiber and nutrients, and some studies have suggested it may have a positive effect on blood sugar control. However, more research is needed to fully understand its benefits.

9. Bilberry:

Bilberry is a berry often touted for its potential benefits for diabetes. It contains compounds called anthocyanins that may have antioxidant and anti-inflammatory properties. Some studies suggest that bilberry might help improve insulin sensitivity and reduce blood sugar levels, but more research is needed to confirm its effects on diabetes management.

10. Fenugreek:

Fenugreek seeds are commonly used in traditional medicine for their potential to lower blood sugar levels. Some research suggests that fenugreek may have a positive impact on insulin sensitivity and glycemic control, but more studies are required to establish its role in diabetes treatment.

11. Gymnema Sylvestre:

Gymnema sylvestre is an herb known for its potential to reduce sugar absorption in the intestines and enhance insulin function. Some studies suggest that gymnema sylvestre may help lower blood sugar levels, but further research is needed to determine its efficacy and safety for diabetes management.

12. Cinnamon:

Cinnamon has been studied for its potential benefits in diabetes management. Some research suggests that cinnamon may improve insulin sensitivity and lower blood sugar levels. While the evidence is promising, the amount of cinnamon required for these effects is higher than what is typically used in culinary amounts.

13. Olive Leaf Extract:

Olive leaf extract contains compounds that may have antioxidant and anti-inflammatory properties. Some studies suggest that it may contribute to improved insulin sensitivity and glycemic control, but more research is needed to establish its role in diabetes treatment.

14. Berberine:

Berberine is a compound found in several plants and has been investigated for its potential effects on blood sugar regulation. Some studies indicate that berberine may help improve insulin sensitivity and reduce blood sugar levels, making it a topic of interest in diabetes research.

15. Licorice Root:

Licorice root is another herb that has been used traditionally and is believed to have potential benefits for diabetes management. Some studies suggest that certain compounds in licorice root may help regulate blood sugar levels, but its long-term safety and effectiveness require further investigation.

16. Consultation with Healthcare Professionals:

It's important to approach the use of herbal remedies for diabetes with caution. While some of the herbs mentioned above may show promise in preliminary studies, more rigorous research is needed to establish their efficacy, optimal dosage, and potential interactions with medications. If you are considering using herbal remedies as part of your diabetes management, it's crucial to consult with a qualified healthcare professional, such as a physician or registered dietitian. They can provide personalized guidance, assess potential risks, and help you make informed decisions about incorporating herbal remedies into your overall diabetes management plan.

The Alkaline Diet for Diabetes Control

The alkaline diet, also known as the alkaline ash diet or acid-alkaline diet, is based on the principle that certain foods can impact the body's pH level, either making it more acidic or more alkaline. Proponents of this diet believe that consuming more alkaline-forming foods can have various health benefits, including better diabetes control. However, it's important to note that the scientific evidence supporting the direct impact of the alkaline diet on diabetes is limited. Let's explore the alkaline diet and its potential implications for diabetes control in detail:

The Alkaline Diet Principles:

The alkaline diet emphasizes consuming foods that are considered alkaline-forming and minimizing foods that are acid-forming. Alkaline-forming foods are typically plant-based, nutrient-dense, and rich in vitamins, minerals, and antioxidants. These foods are believed to help the body maintain a slightly alkaline pH, which proponents suggest can promote overall health.

Foods Typically Included in the Alkaline Diet:

- **Fruits:** Most fruits are considered alkaline-forming, including berries, apples, pears, citrus fruits, and melons.
- **Vegetables:** Leafy greens, cruciferous vegetables (such as broccoli and kale), carrots, beets, and bell peppers are commonly included.
- **Nuts and Seeds:** Almonds, walnuts, flaxseeds, and chia seeds are often included for their healthy fats and protein content.
- **Legumes:** Beans, lentils, and chickpeas are rich in fiber, protein, and essential nutrients.
- **Whole Grains:** Quinoa, millet, brown rice, and oats are preferred over refined grains.
- **Healthy Fats:** Avocado and olive oil are commonly used sources of healthy fats.
- **Herbs and Spices:** Herbs like basil, thyme, and turmeric, as well as spices like ginger and garlic, are often incorporated for flavor and potential health benefits.

Foods Typically Limited in the Alkaline Diet:

1. **Animal Products:** Meat, poultry, and dairy products are generally limited due to their potential to contribute to acidity in the body.
2. **Processed Foods:** Highly processed foods, sugary snacks, and refined grains are discouraged.
3. **Caffeine and Alcohol:** Coffee, tea, and alcohol are often reduced in the alkaline diet.

Potential Implications for Diabetes Control:

While the alkaline diet emphasizes whole, plant-based foods that are generally nutritious, the direct impact of the diet on diabetes control is not well-established. Some proponents of the alkaline diet suggest that it may help with diabetes management by promoting weight loss, reducing inflammation, and improving insulin sensitivity. However, scientific evidence specific to the alkaline diet's effect on diabetes outcomes is limited.

Considerations and Recommendations:

1. **Consultation with Healthcare Professionals:** Before making significant dietary changes, especially if you have diabetes, it's important to consult with a healthcare provider. They can provide personalized guidance based on your individual health needs and conditions.
2. **Balanced Approach:** The alkaline diet's emphasis on whole, nutrient-dense foods aligns with principles of healthy eating. However, it's crucial to maintain a balanced and varied diet that meets your nutritional requirements.
3. **Blood Sugar Monitoring:** If you have diabetes, continue monitoring your blood sugar levels regularly, regardless of dietary changes. This will help you understand how your diet affects your blood sugar and overall health.
4. **Individualized Approach:** Every person's response to different diets can vary. Some individuals may find benefit from incorporating more alkaline-forming foods, while others may not notice significant changes.
5. **Hydration:** Staying properly hydrated is important for overall health, including diabetes management. Drinking water helps maintain optimal bodily functions and supports kidney function, which is especially important for individuals with diabetes.

6. **Portion Control:** Even when following the alkaline diet, portion control is crucial for managing blood sugar levels. Overeating, even with alkaline-forming foods, can lead to spikes in blood sugar.

7. **Whole Foods:** Emphasize whole foods and minimize processed foods, regardless of their alkalinity. Processed foods can contain hidden sugars and unhealthy fats that can affect blood sugar levels.

8. **Monitor Blood Sugar:** Regularly monitor your blood sugar levels to understand how different foods, including alkaline-forming ones, impact your body. This information will help you make informed choices and tailor your diet to your needs.

9. **Individual Variation:** Remember that individual responses to diets can vary. While some people may find benefits from the alkaline diet, others may not experience significant changes in their blood sugar levels.

10. **Consult a Registered Dietitian:** Consider working with a registered dietitian who has expertise in diabetes management. They can help you create a well-balanced meal plan that considers your dietary preferences, health goals, and blood sugar control.

Exercise and Diabetes Management

Exercise is a powerful tool for managing diabetes, regardless of the type. Regular physical activity can help improve insulin sensitivity, lower blood sugar levels, reduce the risk of complications, and enhance overall well-being. Whether you have type 1 diabetes, type 2 diabetes, or are at risk for diabetes, incorporating exercise into your routine can have numerous benefits. Let's delve into the details of how exercise impacts diabetes management:

How Exercise Affects Diabetes:

1. **Improves Insulin Sensitivity:** Exercise enhances the body's sensitivity to insulin, allowing cells to use glucose more effectively for energy. This can lead to better blood sugar control.

2. **Lowers Blood Sugar Levels:** Physical activity helps muscles take up glucose from the bloodstream, leading to a decrease in blood sugar levels. This effect can last even after

you've finished exercising.

3. **Weight Management:** Exercise can aid in weight loss or weight maintenance, which is especially important for type 2 diabetes management. Maintaining a healthy weight contributes to better blood sugar control.

4. **Reduces Cardiovascular Risk:** Regular exercise helps lower the risk of heart disease, a common complication of diabetes. It can improve heart health by reducing blood pressure, cholesterol levels, and inflammation.

5. **Boosts Mood and Mental Health:** Physical activity stimulates the release of endorphins, which are natural mood enhancers. Exercise can reduce stress, anxiety, and depression, promoting overall mental well-being.

6. **Enhances Energy Levels:** Engaging in regular physical activity can increase energy levels and reduce feelings of fatigue, contributing to an improved quality of life.

Exercise Recommendations:

1. **Aerobic Exercise:** Activities such as brisk walking, jogging, cycling, swimming, and dancing are excellent choices for improving cardiovascular health and blood sugar control. Aim for at least 150 minutes of moderate-intensity aerobic exercise per week, spread across several days.

2. **Strength Training:** Incorporate strength training exercises like weightlifting, resistance bands, or bodyweight exercises. Building muscle mass can enhance insulin sensitivity and metabolism. Include these activities on at least two days per week.

3. **Flexibility and Balance:** Practices like yoga and tai chi can help improve flexibility, balance, and relaxation. These activities support overall well-being and can be incorporated regularly.

Exercise and Blood Sugar Monitoring:

If you have diabetes, it's crucial to monitor your blood sugar levels before, during, and after exercise. This helps you understand how different types and durations of physical activity affect your blood sugar. Monitoring allows you to adjust your insulin or oral medication doses, if needed, and prevent both hypoglycemia (low blood sugar) and hyperglycemia (high blood sugar).

Precautions and Considerations:

1. **Consult a Healthcare Professional:** Before starting a new exercise regimen, consult your healthcare provider, especially if you have any underlying health conditions.
2. **Individualized Approach:** The type and intensity of exercise that suits you will depend on your fitness level, health status, and preferences.
3. **Hydration:** Stay hydrated before, during, and after exercise to avoid dehydration.
4. **Snacking:** Have a small carbohydrate-containing snack if your blood sugar is low before exercising to prevent hypoglycemia.
5. **Foot Care:** Pay attention to foot health, especially if you have diabetes-related neuropathy. Wear appropriate footwear and check your feet regularly.
6. **Monitor Responses:** Pay attention to how your body responds to different activities. If you experience unusual symptoms or significant changes in blood sugar levels, consult your healthcare provider.

Tips for Successful Exercise and Diabetes Management:

1. **Start Slowly:** If you're new to exercise or have been inactive for a while, start with gentle activities and gradually increase intensity and duration.
2. **Warm-Up and Cool-Down:** Always begin with a warm-up to prepare your body for exercise and end with a cool-down to help your heart rate return to normal.
3. **Set Realistic Goals:** Set achievable fitness goals that align with your current fitness level and health status. Celebrate your progress along the way.
4. **Variety:** Mix up your exercise routine to prevent boredom and engage different muscle groups. This can also help you stay motivated.
5. **Consistency:** Aim for regular exercise rather than sporadic intense workouts. Consistency is more important for long-term benefits.
6. **Listen to Your Body:** If you feel unwell or experience symptoms like dizziness, nausea, or extreme fatigue during exercise, stop and consult a healthcare professional.
7. **Hypos and Hypers:** Be prepared for potential low blood sugar (hypoglycemia) during or after exercise. Have a fast-acting carbohydrate source on hand in case your blood sugar drops.

8. **Stay Safe:** If you're on insulin or medications that lower blood sugar, monitor your levels before and after exercise to prevent dangerous drops in blood sugar.

9. **Stay Informed:** Keep learning about diabetes management and exercise. Understanding how your body responds to different activities will help you make informed choices.

10. **Adapt and Adjust:** Your exercise needs may change over time, so be willing to adapt your routine as your fitness level and health status evolve.

Living Well with Diabetes: Empowering a Healthy Lifestyle

Living well with diabetes involves adopting a holistic approach to health that encompasses not only medical management but also lifestyle choices, emotional well-being, and self-empowerment. With the right strategies and mindset, individuals with diabetes can lead fulfilling lives while effectively managing their condition. Let's explore how to empower a healthy lifestyle while living with diabetes:

1. Education and Awareness:

Understanding diabetes is essential for effective management. Educate yourself about the different types of diabetes, blood sugar monitoring, medications, complications, and lifestyle modifications. Staying informed empowers you to make informed decisions and collaborate with your healthcare team.

2. Balanced Nutrition:

Adopting a balanced and healthy diet is crucial. Focus on whole, nutrient-rich foods like fruits, vegetables, lean proteins, whole grains, and healthy fats. Monitor carbohydrate intake to help manage blood sugar levels. Working with a registered dietitian can provide personalized guidance.

3. Regular Physical Activity:

Incorporate regular exercise into your routine, following your healthcare provider's recommendations. Engage in activities you enjoy, such as walking, cycling, swimming, or dancing. Aim for a combination of aerobic, strength, and flexibility exercises.

4. Blood Sugar Monitoring:

Regularly monitor your blood sugar levels as directed by your healthcare provider. This helps you understand how your lifestyle choices, including diet and exercise, impact your blood sugar levels.

5. Medication Adherence:

If you're prescribed medications, follow your healthcare provider's instructions diligently. Take medications as prescribed, and communicate any concerns or side effects to your provider.

6. Stress Management:

Chronic stress can affect blood sugar levels. Practice stress-reduction techniques like meditation, deep breathing, yoga, or mindfulness to promote emotional well-being.

7. Sleep Quality:

Prioritize getting adequate and restful sleep. Poor sleep can affect blood sugar control and overall health. Maintain a regular sleep schedule and create a relaxing bedtime routine.

8. Support System:

Build a strong support network that includes family, friends, healthcare providers, and support groups. Connecting with others who understand your journey can provide emotional support and practical advice.

9. Regular Check-Ups:

Attend regular check-ups with your healthcare provider. These appointments help monitor your diabetes, assess your overall health, and make any necessary adjustments to your management plan.

10. Self-Advocacy:

Be an active participant in your healthcare. Ask questions, express your concerns, and collaborate with your healthcare team to make decisions that align with your health goals.

11. Problem-Solving:

Diabetes management can present challenges. Develop problem-solving skills to address issues that arise, whether related to blood sugar fluctuations, meal planning, or physical activity.

12. Positive Mindset:

Maintain a positive attitude and focus on your strengths. A positive mindset can influence your ability to cope with challenges and make healthy choices.

13. Embrace Flexibility:

Life can be unpredictable. Embrace flexibility in your management plan and adapt to changes while staying committed to your overall health goals.

14. Celebrate Achievements:

Celebrate your successes, whether big or small. Recognize your efforts and achievements in managing your diabetes and making positive lifestyle changes.

15. Seek Professional Help:

If you're struggling with emotional or mental health challenges, seek support from mental health professionals. Managing diabetes involves not only physical well-being but also emotional well-being.

16. Mindful Eating:

Practice mindful eating by paying attention to your hunger and fullness cues. Avoid overeating and make conscious food choices that align with your health goals.

17. Hydration:

Stay hydrated by drinking plenty of water throughout the day. Proper hydration supports overall bodily functions and can help regulate blood sugar levels.

18. Meal Planning:

Plan your meals and snacks in advance to help manage your blood sugar levels. Consistency in meal timing and portion control can contribute to stable blood sugar.

19. Limit Alcohol Intake:

If you choose to consume alcohol, do so in moderation and be mindful of its impact on blood sugar levels. Alcohol can affect blood sugar regulation and interact with medications.

20. Travel Preparedness:

If you're traveling, plan ahead by ensuring you have access to necessary supplies, medications, and snacks. Consult your healthcare provider for guidance on managing your diabetes while traveling.

21. Embrace New Technologies:

Explore technological advancements such as continuous glucose monitoring (CGM) systems and insulin pumps. These tools can provide valuable insights into your blood sugar trends and improve your diabetes management.

22. Celebrate Progress, Not Perfection:

Remember that managing diabetes is a journey. Focus on progress rather than aiming for perfection. Celebrate your achievements and stay motivated to continue making positive changes.

23. Avoid Comparisons:

Your diabetes journey is unique to you. Avoid comparing your progress to others. What works for one person may not work for another, so focus on your individual goals and needs.

24. Adapt to Life Changes:

Life is full of changes, and your diabetes management may need adjustments along the way. Whether it's changes in medication, routines, or lifestyle, be open to adapting and seeking guidance when needed.

25. Maintain a Positive Outlook:

Cultivate a positive outlook on life. Surround yourself with positivity, engage in activities you enjoy, and practice gratitude. A positive mindset can enhance your overall well-being.

26. Set Realistic Goals:

Set achievable health and lifestyle goals that are specific, measurable, attainable, relevant, and time-bound (SMART). Regularly review and adjust your goals as needed.

27. Stay Informed:

Stay up-to-date with the latest developments in diabetes management, treatments, and research. Being informed empowers you to make educated decisions about your health.

28. Share Your Story:

Sharing your diabetes journey with others can raise awareness, reduce stigma, and inspire others facing similar challenges. Your experiences can make a positive impact on others' lives.

Conclusion:

Living well with diabetes is about finding a balance that suits your unique needs, preferences, and health goals. By incorporating these strategies and embracing a holistic approach to diabetes management, you can navigate the challenges, make informed choices, and lead a fulfilling life. Remember that you have the power to take control of your diabetes and live a healthy and empowered lifestyle. Your journey is ongoing, and with the right tools, support, and determination, you can thrive while effectively managing your diabetes.

Book 6: Lupus Unraveled: Dr. Sebi's Natural Treatment for Lupus

Understanding Lupus: Types and Symptoms

Lupus, also known as systemic lupus erythematosus (SLE), is a complex autoimmune disease that can affect various parts of the body. It often presents with a wide range of symptoms and can vary significantly from person to person. Understanding the different types of lupus and their associated symptoms is crucial for early diagnosis and effective management. Let's delve into the details of lupus types and their symptoms:

1. Systemic Lupus Erythematosus (SLE):

Description: SLE is the most common form of lupus and can affect multiple systems in the body, including skin, joints, kidneys, heart, lungs, brain, and blood cells.

Symptoms: The symptoms of SLE can be diverse and may include:

- Fatigue and weakness
- Joint pain and stiffness
- Skin rashes, such as the classic butterfly rash on the face
- Fever
- Photosensitivity (sensitivity to sunlight)
- Mouth or nose sores
- Hair loss
- Raynaud's phenomenon (color changes in fingers and toes in response to cold)
- Chest pain or discomfort
- Kidney problems
- Cognitive difficulties, including memory issues and confusion

2. Cutaneous Lupus Erythematosus (CLE):

- **Description:** CLE primarily affects the skin and is divided into different subtypes, including discoid lupus erythematosus (DLE) and subacute cutaneous lupus erythematosus (SCLE).
- **Symptoms:**
  - DLE: Raised, scaly red patches or plaques on the skin, often on the face and scalp.

These can lead to scarring and skin discoloration.

- ○ SCLE: Rash with raised, scaly patches that are often worsened by sun exposure. The rash typically appears on areas exposed to sunlight.

3. Drug-Induced Lupus Erythematosus (DIL):

- **Description:** DIL is triggered by certain medications and typically resolves once the medication is discontinued.
- **Symptoms:** Similar to SLE but generally milder, symptoms may include joint pain, rash, fever, and muscle pain. Kidney and central nervous system involvement is rare in DIL.

4. Neonatal Lupus:

- **Description:** Neonatal lupus occurs when a mother's autoantibodies affect her newborn. It's usually temporary and does not result in long-term health issues for the baby.
- **Symptoms:** Rash, liver problems, and, in some cases, heart block in the baby's heart rhythm. Symptoms usually disappear within a few months.

5. Other Types of Lupus:

- **Lupus Nephritis:** Kidney inflammation is a common complication of SLE and can lead to various kidney-related symptoms, including swelling, high blood pressure, and changes in urine.
- **Central Nervous System Lupus:** Inflammation of the brain and spinal cord can lead to symptoms such as headaches, seizures, mood changes, and cognitive difficulties.
- **Cardiovascular Lupus:** Lupus can increase the risk of cardiovascular issues such as heart disease, inflammation of the heart lining, and other cardiac complications.

Diagnosis and Monitoring:

- **Laboratory Tests:** Blood tests for markers like antinuclear antibodies (ANA), anti-dsDNA antibodies, and anti-Smith antibodies are used to assist in diagnosing lupus. These tests help identify autoimmune activity and can aid in differentiating lupus from other conditions.
- **Complete Blood Count (CBC):** Measures red and white blood cells and platelets,

helping to detect anemia, low white blood cell counts, and low platelet counts that may occur in lupus.

- **Kidney Function Tests:** Blood and urine tests can assess kidney function and detect signs of kidney inflammation, crucial in cases of lupus nephritis.
- **Imaging:** X-rays, ultrasound, and other imaging tests may be used to examine joints and organs, especially in cases of suspected joint or organ involvement.
- **Skin Biopsy:** In cases of cutaneous lupus, a skin biopsy may be performed to examine tissue under a microscope and confirm the diagnosis.

Treatment and Management:

- **Medications:** Treatment often involves a combination of medications based on symptoms and disease severity. Common medications include:
  - o Nonsteroidal anti-inflammatory drugs (NSAIDs) for joint pain and inflammation.
  - o Antimalarial drugs, such as hydroxychloroquine, for skin and joint symptoms.
  - o Corticosteroids to manage inflammation during flares.
  - o Immunosuppressive drugs to suppress the immune system and reduce autoimmune activity.
  - o Biologic therapies, such as monoclonal antibodies, for severe cases.
- **Lifestyle Modifications:** Adopting a healthy lifestyle can complement medical treatment:
  - Protecting your skin from sunlight and using sunscreen to prevent worsening of skin symptoms.
  - Managing stress through relaxation techniques, exercise, and mindfulness.
  - Regular exercise to maintain joint mobility, strength, and overall well-being.
- **Regular Monitoring:** Lupus is a chronic condition that requires ongoing monitoring by healthcare professionals. Regular check-ups, blood tests, and communication with your medical team are essential to adjust treatments as needed and monitor disease activity.

Emotional and Mental Health:

- **Support Groups:** Connecting with others who share similar experiences can provide emotional support and valuable insights.
- **Therapy and Counseling:** Therapists or counselors can help you manage the emotional challenges associated with living with lupus.

- **Educational Resources:** Learning about lupus and becoming informed about your condition can empower you to make informed decisions and advocate for your health.

Dr. Sebi's Herbal Recommendations for Lupus

Dr. Sebi, also known as Alfredo Darrington Bowman, was a Honduran herbalist and self-proclaimed healer who advocated for natural healing methods and promoted the use of plant-based diets and herbal remedies for various health conditions, including lupus. It's important to note that Dr. Sebi's recommendations and claims are not supported by mainstream medical authorities and lack scientific validation. Before considering any alternative treatments, including those suggested by Dr. Sebi, it's advisable to consult with a qualified healthcare professional. With that in mind, let's explore some of the herbal recommendations that Dr. Sebi proposed for lupus:

1. Irish Moss (Sea Moss):

Dr. Sebi often recommended Irish moss, a type of seaweed, for various health conditions, including lupus. He claimed that Irish moss could help cleanse the body and provide essential nutrients. However, there is limited scientific evidence supporting Irish moss as a specific treatment for lupus.

2. Bladderwrack:

Bladderwrack is another seaweed that Dr. Sebi often mentioned. He believed that it could contribute to detoxification and overall health. While bladderwrack does contain minerals and nutrients, its effectiveness in treating lupus has not been established through rigorous scientific research.

3. Burdock Root:

Dr. Sebi frequently recommended burdock root for its potential cleansing and detoxifying properties. Burdock root is known for its potential diuretic and anti-inflammatory effects, but its specific role in managing lupus is not supported by robust scientific evidence.

4. Dandelion:

Dandelion is a plant often suggested for its potential benefits in supporting liver health and detoxification. Dr. Sebi believed that dandelion could aid in purifying the body, but its role in treating lupus is not substantiated by scientific studies.

5. Sarsaparilla:

Sarsaparilla root was mentioned by Dr. Sebi as a remedy for various health conditions, including lupus. While sarsaparilla has been used traditionally in herbal medicine, its specific effects on lupus are not well-documented in scientific literature.

6. Irish Seamoss and Bladderwrack Mix:

Dr. Sebi often recommended a mixture of Irish moss and bladderwrack as part of his approach to health and wellness. He claimed that this combination could provide essential nutrients and support overall well-being.

7. Elimination of Processed Foods:

Dr. Sebi advocated for a plant-based diet that excludes processed foods, refined sugars, and artificial additives. He believed that this dietary approach could contribute to improved health and the management of various conditions, including lupus.

8. Alkaline Diet:

Dr. Sebi emphasized an alkaline diet, which consists of consuming mostly alkaline-forming foods to maintain a balanced pH level in the body. He believed that an alkaline diet could support overall health and help manage various health issues.

9. Yellow Dock:

Yellow dock is another herb that Dr. Sebi suggested for various health conditions, including lupus. It's believed to have detoxifying properties and is often used in traditional herbal medicine. However, its specific role in managing lupus is not supported by strong scientific evidence.

10. Red Clover:

Dr. Sebi occasionally mentioned red clover as a potential herbal remedy. Red clover is known for its potential phytoestrogenic and antioxidant effects. While it has been used in traditional medicine for various purposes, its direct impact on lupus management is not well-established.

11. Lily of the Valley:

Lily of the valley is a plant that Dr. Sebi sometimes recommended. It's traditionally used for its potential cardiovascular benefits. However, there is no substantial scientific evidence linking lily of the valley to lupus treatment.

12. Consultation with Healthcare Professionals:

Before considering any of Dr. Sebi's herbal recommendations or alternative treatments for lupus, it's essential to consult with a qualified healthcare professional. Lupus is a complex autoimmune disease that requires a comprehensive medical approach. Your healthcare provider can offer guidance, recommend evidence-based treatments, and help you make informed decisions about incorporating herbal remedies into your lupus management plan.

Adopting an Alkaline Diet for Lupus Management

The alkaline diet is based on the concept that certain foods can impact the body's pH level, potentially affecting health and well-being. While proponents of the alkaline diet claim various benefits, including improved immune function and reduced inflammation, it's important to note that the scientific evidence supporting the direct impact of the alkaline diet on lupus management is limited. However, adopting a balanced and nutrient-rich diet can contribute to overall well-being, which is especially important for individuals with lupus. Let's explore the alkaline diet in the context of lupus management:

The Alkaline Diet Principles:

The alkaline diet focuses on consuming foods that are believed to have an alkalizing effect on the body, helping to maintain a slightly alkaline pH. This diet emphasizes plant-based foods, including fruits, vegetables, nuts, seeds, legumes, and whole grains. It also encourages minimizing or avoiding acid-forming foods like meat, dairy, refined sugar, processed foods, and caffeine.

Potential Benefits for Lupus Management:

While there is limited scientific evidence directly linking the alkaline diet to lupus management, some aspects of the diet may be beneficial:

1. **Nutrient-Rich Foods:** The alkaline diet promotes the consumption of nutrient-dense foods, such as fruits and vegetables, which are rich in vitamins, minerals, antioxidants, and phytochemicals. These nutrients can support overall health and immune function.

2. **Anti-Inflammatory Potential:** Some alkaline-forming foods, such as leafy greens and berries, are known for their potential anti-inflammatory properties. Inflammation is a key component of lupus, so consuming foods that may reduce inflammation could be beneficial.

3. **Hydration:** The diet encourages drinking plenty of water, which is essential for maintaining optimal bodily functions and supporting kidney health, an important consideration for individuals with lupus.

4. **Balanced Approach:** The emphasis on whole foods aligns with general healthy eating

principles, which can contribute to overall well-being, weight management, and cardiovascular health.

Considerations and Recommendations:

1. **Consultation with Healthcare Professionals:** Before making significant dietary changes, consult your healthcare provider, especially if you have lupus. Your healthcare team can provide personalized guidance based on your individual health needs and condition.

2. **Balanced Nutrition:** While the alkaline diet promotes many healthy foods, it's important to maintain a balanced and varied diet to ensure you're getting all the essential nutrients your body needs.

3. **Individualized Approach:** Each person's experience with lupus is unique. Some individuals may find certain dietary changes beneficial, while others may not notice significant effects.

4. **Blood Sugar Monitoring:** If you have lupus and diabetes, be mindful of the impact of the alkaline diet on your blood sugar levels. Regular monitoring is essential.

5. **Medication and Treatment:** The alkaline diet should not be used as a replacement for prescribed medications and treatments for lupus. Continue to follow your healthcare provider's recommendations.

5. Alkaline Diet and Medication:

It's important to note that the alkaline diet should not be considered a replacement for prescribed medications for lupus. Lupus is a complex autoimmune condition that requires comprehensive medical management. Any dietary changes, including adopting an alkaline diet, should be discussed with your healthcare provider to ensure they are safe and appropriate for your individual health needs.

6. Potential Challenges:

While the alkaline diet emphasizes many nutrient-rich foods, it may also present challenges:

- **Dietary Restriction:** The diet restricts certain foods, which could lead to potential nutrient deficiencies if not carefully planned.

- **Social and Practical Considerations:** Following the diet might be challenging in social situations or when dining out.
- **Variety and Balance:** Focusing exclusively on alkaline-forming foods might limit dietary variety and lead to an imbalance in essential nutrients.

7. Blood Sugar Management:

For individuals with lupus and diabetes, the alkaline diet's potential impact on blood sugar levels should be considered. Some alkaline-forming foods, such as fruits and starchy vegetables, can affect blood sugar. Monitoring blood sugar levels and consulting with a registered dietitian or healthcare provider are important steps.

8. Working with a Registered Dietitian:

If you're considering adopting an alkaline diet for lupus management, working with a registered dietitian who specializes in autoimmune conditions can provide valuable guidance. They can help you create a balanced meal plan that meets your nutritional needs while also addressing the specific challenges of lupus.

9. Listening to Your Body:

Every individual's response to dietary changes can vary. Pay attention to how your body reacts to different foods and make adjustments as needed. If you experience any adverse effects or changes in symptoms, consult your healthcare provider.

10. Holistic Approach:

While the alkaline diet is one aspect of a healthy lifestyle, it's important to approach lupus management holistically. Focus on a combination of evidence-based medical treatments, regular exercise, stress management, sleep, and emotional well-being.

Managing Emotional Wellbeing with Lupus

Living with lupus can bring about a range of emotional challenges due to the physical symptoms, unpredictable nature of the disease, and the impact it can have on daily life. Managing your emotional well-being is essential for maintaining a positive quality of life while effectively managing your health. Here's a comprehensive guide on how to address emotional well-being when living with lupus:

Understanding Emotional Challenges:

1. **Anxiety and Stress:** The uncertainty of lupus, managing symptoms, and potential flares can contribute to heightened anxiety and stress levels.
2. **Depression:** Chronic illness, pain, and limitations can lead to feelings of sadness and depression.
3. **Grief and Loss:** Lupus may require adjustments to lifestyle, hobbies, and social activities, leading to a sense of loss and grief.
4. **Isolation:** Fluctuating energy levels and potential mobility challenges can lead to social isolation and feelings of loneliness.

Thriving with Lupus: Embracing a Life Beyond the Diagnosis

Receiving a lupus diagnosis can be a life-changing event, but it doesn't mean giving up on living a fulfilling and meaningful life. Thriving with lupus involves embracing a holistic approach that goes beyond the challenges of the disease and focuses on personal growth, well-being, and pursuing your passions. Here's a comprehensive guide on how to thrive while living with lupus:

1. Shift Your Perspective:

- **Mindset Matters:** Cultivate a positive mindset that acknowledges challenges but also focuses on opportunities, growth, and resilience.
- **Reframe Challenges:** View obstacles as opportunities for personal development and learning. Find lessons and strengths within adversity.

2. Self-Care and Prioritization:

- **Health Comes First:** Prioritize self-care, including managing your health, getting adequate rest, and following medical advice.
- **Healthy Lifestyle:** Incorporate a balanced diet, regular exercise, and stress management into your routine to support overall well-being.

3. Set Realistic Goals:

- **Dream Big:** Set ambitious but achievable goals that align with your passions and interests.
- **Break It Down:** Divide larger goals into smaller, manageable steps to avoid feeling overwhelmed.

4. Pursue Your Passions:

- **Find Joy:** Engage in activities that bring you joy and fulfillment, whether it's a hobby, creative pursuit, or volunteering.
- **Creativity:** Express yourself through creative outlets like art, music, writing, or crafts.

5. Adapt and Adjust:

- **Flexibility:** Understand that life with lupus may require adjustments. Be open to changing plans and finding alternative routes to your goals.
- **Problem-Solving:** Develop problem-solving skills to address challenges creatively and proactively.

6. Social Support:

- **Connect:** Build and nurture relationships with friends, family, and supportive communities.
- **Share Your Story:** Sharing your lupus journey can inspire others and create a sense of purpose.

7. Mindfulness and Acceptance:

- **Stay Present:** Practice mindfulness to stay present and focused on the current moment, reducing stress and anxiety.

- **Acceptance:** Embrace your journey, acknowledging that lupus is a part of your life but not defining your entire identity.

8. Educate Yourself:

- **Empowerment:** Knowledge is power. Educate yourself about lupus to make informed decisions and advocate for your health.

9. Manage Stress:

- **Stress Reduction:** Practice stress-reduction techniques such as meditation, deep breathing, and yoga to manage stressors.
- **Self-Compassion:** Be kind to yourself and avoid putting undue pressure on yourself.

10. Seek Professional Support:

- **Therapeutic Help:** If needed, seek guidance from therapists or counselors to navigate emotional challenges.

11. Celebrate Achievements:

- **Acknowledge Progress:** Celebrate your achievements and milestones, no matter how small. Each step forward is a victory.

12. Embrace Gratitude:

- **Gratitude Practice:** Cultivate a practice of gratitude, focusing on the positive aspects of your life and experiences.

13. Advocate for Yourself:

- **Be Your Advocate:** Speak up for your needs and priorities in healthcare settings. Be an active participant in your treatment plan.

14. Practice Resilience:

- **Build Resilience:** Develop the ability to bounce back from challenges and setbacks. Resilience is a key trait in thriving with a chronic condition like lupus.

- **Learn from Setbacks:** Instead of dwelling on setbacks, use them as opportunities to learn and grow stronger.

15. Embrace Independence:

- **Empowerment:** Take control of your health and decisions, while also recognizing when you need assistance.
- **Set Boundaries:** Establish boundaries to avoid overexerting yourself and maintain your well-being.

16. Explore New Horizons:

- **Continual Growth:** Seek opportunities for personal growth, learning, and expanding your horizons.
- **Explore Interests:** Try new activities or hobbies that align with your passions and bring a sense of accomplishment.

17. Nurture Relationships:

- **Connection:** Foster meaningful relationships that provide emotional support, understanding, and companionship.
- **Effective Communication:** Clearly communicate your needs, challenges, and victories with your loved ones.

18. Celebrate Self-Care:

- **Regular Self-Care:** Dedicate time to self-care activities that nurture your physical, emotional, and mental well-being.
- **Unplug:** Disconnect from electronic devices and create quiet moments to recharge.

19. Be Patient with Yourself:

- **Practice Patience:** Understand that progress takes time. Be patient with yourself as you navigate challenges and make changes.
- **Self-Compassion:** Treat yourself with kindness and understanding, especially during difficult times.

20. Embrace Uncertainty:

- **Adaptability:** Develop adaptability to cope with the unpredictability of lupus. Embrace the ebb and flow of life.

21. Set Healthy Boundaries:

- **Protect Your Energy:** Recognize when to say no to commitments that drain your energy and negatively impact your health.

22. Cultivate Meaning:

- **Purpose and Meaning:** Find purpose and meaning in everyday activities, relationships, and pursuing your goals.

23. Reflect and Adjust:

- **Periodic Reflection:** Take time to reflect on your journey, celebrate achievements, and adjust your goals as needed.

24. Focus on What You Can Control:

- **Empowerment:** Concentrate on aspects of your life that you can control and influence, rather than dwelling on circumstances beyond your control.

25. Holistic Well-Being:

- **Balance:** Strive for a holistic approach to well-being that encompasses physical, emotional, mental, and social health.

Book 7: Healthy Hair, Naturally: Dr. Sebi's Guide to Preventing Hair Loss

Understanding Hair Loss: Causes and Types

Hair loss, also known as alopecia, is a common concern that affects people of all ages and genders. It can have various causes and manifest in different ways. Understanding the underlying factors and types of hair loss is crucial for effectively addressing the condition. Let's explore the causes and types of hair loss in detail:

Causes of Hair Loss:

1. Androgenetic Alopecia (Male and Female Pattern Baldness):

- **Description:** This is the most common cause of hair loss and is influenced by genetics and hormones.
- **Symptoms:** Gradual thinning of hair, receding hairline in men, and widening part in women.
- **Causes:** Hormones (specifically dihydrotestosterone), genetic predisposition, and age.

2. Telogen Effluvium:

- **Description:** This type of hair loss is usually temporary and occurs due to a disruption in the hair growth cycle.
- **Symptoms:** Sudden diffuse shedding of hair, often following a significant event like surgery, illness, childbirth, or emotional stress.
- **Causes:** Physical or emotional stressors that push a larger percentage of hairs into the resting (telogen) phase, leading to shedding a few months later.

3. Alopecia Areata:

- **Description:** An autoimmune condition that causes sudden hair loss in distinct patches.
- **Symptoms:** Circular or oval patches of hair loss, typically on the scalp but can affect other body hair as well.
- **Causes:** Autoimmune response targeting hair follicles, possibly triggered by genetics and environmental factors.

4. Traction Alopecia:

- **Description:** Hair loss due to repeated pulling or tension on the hair shafts.
- **Symptoms:** Hair loss along the hairline, especially from tight hairstyles (braids, ponytails) or excessive use of hair extensions.
- **Causes:** Constant tension weakens hair follicles, leading to hair breakage and loss.

5. Trichotillomania:

- **Description:** A psychological disorder characterized by the urge to pull out one's hair.
- **Symptoms:** Patchy hair loss due to repeated hair pulling, often leading to noticeable bald spots.
- **Causes:** Emotional distress and impulse control issues.

6. Medical Conditions and Treatments:

- **Description:** Various medical conditions and treatments can lead to hair loss.
- **Symptoms:** Hair loss as a secondary symptom of underlying health conditions, such as thyroid disorders, autoimmune diseases, and certain medications like chemotherapy.
- **Causes:** Underlying medical issues or side effects of treatments affecting hair follicles.

Types of Hair Loss:

1. Androgenetic Alopecia:

- **Description:** Gradual thinning of hair in predictable patterns, often hereditary.
- **Affected Areas:** Scalp in both men and women.

2. Alopecia Areata:

- **Description:** Sudden onset of well-defined bald patches.
- **Affected Areas:** Scalp and other body hair.

3. Telogen Effluvium:

- **Description:** Temporary hair shedding due to stress or hormonal changes.
- **Affected Areas:** Scalp.

4. Traction Alopecia:

- **Description:** Hair loss due to repeated tension on hair follicles.
- **Affected Areas:** Primarily around the hairline and where tension is applied.

5. Trichotillomania:

- **Description:** Hair loss due to compulsive hair pulling.
- **Affected Areas:** Any area of the body with hair.

6. Anagen Effluvium:

- **Description:** Sudden hair loss due to disruption of the anagen (growth) phase of the hair cycle.
- **Affected Areas:** Scalp and other body hair.
- **Causes:** Often associated with chemotherapy or exposure to toxic substances.

Diagnosis and Evaluation:

- **Medical History:** A healthcare provider will gather information about your medical history, family history of hair loss, and any recent events or changes that might have triggered the hair loss.
- **Physical Examination:** A dermatologist will examine your scalp and hair to assess the pattern of hair loss, the condition of the scalp, and any accompanying symptoms.
- **Blood Tests:** Blood tests may be conducted to check for underlying medical conditions that could be causing or contributing to hair loss, such as thyroid disorders or nutritional deficiencies.
- **Pull Test:** A small amount of hair is gently pulled to see how many hairs come out. An increased number of pulled-out hairs can indicate a shedding problem.
- **Scalp Biopsy:** In some cases, a small piece of the scalp may be biopsied to determine the type of hair loss and its underlying cause.

Treatment Options:

- **Topical Treatments:** Medications applied directly to the scalp, such as minoxidil, can stimulate hair growth and slow down hair loss.
- **Oral Medications:** Prescription medications like finasteride may be used to block the effects of hormones that contribute to hair loss.

- **Corticosteroid Injections:** Injections of corticosteroids into the scalp can help reduce inflammation and stimulate hair growth in certain types of alopecia.
- **Hair Transplant:** For individuals with advanced hair loss, hair transplant surgery involves moving hair follicles from one part of the body to areas with thinning or no hair.
- **Laser Therapy:** Low-level laser therapy (LLLT) devices can stimulate hair follicles and promote hair growth.
- **Wigs and Hairpieces:** For temporary or more extensive hair loss, wigs, hairpieces, or hair extensions can provide a cosmetic solution.
- **Psychological Support:** Hair loss can have emotional and psychological effects. Seeking support from therapists or support groups can help individuals cope with the emotional impact of hair loss.

Prevention and Maintenance:

- **Healthy Lifestyle:** A balanced diet rich in nutrients, regular exercise, and stress management contribute to overall well-being and hair health.
- **Gentle Hair Care:** Avoid harsh treatments, excessive heat, and tight hairstyles that can damage hair and contribute to hair loss.
- **Early Intervention:** Addressing hair loss early on can improve the effectiveness of treatments and prevent further hair loss.
- **Medical Management:** If hair loss is linked to an underlying medical condition, proper management of that condition can help prevent or minimize hair loss.

Dr. Sebi's Herbal Remedies for Hair Loss

Dr. Sebi, whose full name is Alfredo Darrington Bowman, was a self-proclaimed herbalist and healer known for promoting natural remedies and a holistic approach to health and wellness. He developed a dietary and lifestyle regimen that focused on alkaline foods and herbal supplements to support overall well-being, including addressing hair loss. Keep in mind that while many people have reported positive experiences with Dr. Sebi's approach, scientific evidence for its effectiveness may be limited. Here are some herbal remedies that Dr. Sebi recommended for hair loss:

1. Burdock Root (Arctium lappa):

- **Benefits:** Burdock root is believed to support hair health by improving blood circulation to the scalp and providing essential nutrients.
- **Usage:** It can be consumed as a tea or in capsule form. It's also available as a tincture.

2. Irish Moss (Chondrus crispus):

- **Benefits**: Irish moss is rich in minerals and nutrients that may contribute to hair health and growth.
- Usage: Irish moss can be consumed as a gel, added to smoothies, or included in other recipes.

3. Bladderwrack (Fucus vesiculosus):

- **Benefits:** Bladderwrack is a type of seaweed that is considered nutrient-dense and may provide essential minerals for hair health.
- **Usage:** Bladderwrack can be consumed as a supplement or added to foods as a seasoning.

4. Nettle (Urtica dioica):

- **Benefits:** Nettle is believed to support hair growth by improving blood circulation to the scalp and providing nutrients.
- **Usage:** Nettle can be consumed as a tea, taken in capsule form, or used topically as a hair rinse.

5. Horsetail (Equisetum arvense):

- **Benefits:** Horsetail contains silica, which is believed to contribute to hair strength and structure.
- **Usage:** Horsetail can be consumed as a tea or taken in capsule form.

6. Aloe Vera (Aloe barbadensis miller):

- **Benefits:** Aloe vera has soothing properties that can help maintain a healthy scalp environment.

- **Usage:** Aloe vera gel can be applied topically to the scalp or consumed as a drink.

7. Sea Moss (Chondrus crispus):

- **Benefits:** Similar to Irish moss, sea moss is rich in minerals that can support overall health and potentially hair growth.
- **Usage:** Sea moss can be consumed as a gel or included in various recipes.

8. Saw Palmetto (Serenoa repens):

- **Benefits:** Saw palmetto is often associated with supporting hormonal balance, which can impact hair health.
- **Usage:** Saw palmetto supplements are available in various forms, including capsules.

9. Chaparral (Larrea tridentata):

- **Benefits:** Chaparral is believed to have detoxifying properties that may contribute to overall health, which could indirectly support hair health.
- **Usage:** Chaparral is available as a supplement, tea, or tincture.

10. Sage (Salvia officinalis):

- **Benefits:** Sage has been used traditionally for its potential benefits for hair and scalp health.
- **Usage:** Sage can be used as a hair rinse, tea, or included in cooking.

Note: Before using any herbal remedies, it's important to consult a healthcare professional or herbalist, especially if you have underlying health conditions, are taking medications, or are pregnant or breastfeeding. Herbal remedies can interact with medications and have varying effects on different individuals.

The Alkaline Diet for Healthy Hair

The alkaline diet is a dietary approach that emphasizes consuming foods that promote an alkaline environment in the body, which is believed to have various health benefits, including supporting healthy hair. The diet primarily consists of alkaline-forming foods such as fruits, vegetables, nuts, seeds, and whole grains, while minimizing acid-forming foods like processed foods, animal products, and refined sugars. Let's delve into how the alkaline diet may contribute to healthy hair:

1. Nutrient-Rich Foods:

- **Fruits and Vegetables:** These foods are rich in vitamins, minerals, antioxidants, and phytochemicals that are essential for overall health, including hair health.
- **Dark Leafy Greens:** Spinach, kale, and Swiss chard are excellent sources of iron, which supports hair growth and strength.
- **Colorful Fruits:** Berries, citrus fruits, and melons provide vitamin C, which helps in the absorption of iron and promotes collagen production, crucial for hair structure.

2. Hydration:

- **Water-Rich Foods:** Many alkaline-forming foods, such as fruits and vegetables, have high water content, contributing to overall hydration, which is important for healthy hair.

3. Nutrient Balance:

- **Essential Fatty Acids:** Nuts, seeds, and certain oils in the alkaline diet provide essential fatty acids that promote scalp health and prevent dryness.
- **Protein Sources:** Plant-based proteins like beans, lentils, quinoa, and nuts contribute to hair structure and growth.

4. Reduced Inflammatory Foods:

- **Processed Foods:** The alkaline diet discourages processed foods high in refined sugars, unhealthy fats, and additives, which can contribute to inflammation that may affect hair health.

- **Acidic Foods:** The diet minimizes acid-forming foods, which some believe can create an environment conducive to inflammation.

5. Improved Digestion:

- **High Fiber:** Alkaline foods often have high fiber content, which supports gut health and efficient nutrient absorption that can benefit hair.

6. Antioxidant Protection:

- **Antioxidant-Rich Foods:** Alkaline foods like berries, leafy greens, and nuts contain antioxidants that protect hair follicles from damage caused by oxidative stress.

7. Alkaline-Forming Foods:

- **Leafy Greens:** Spinach, kale, collard greens, and Swiss chard are highly alkaline and nutrient-dense.
- **Colorful Vegetables:** Bell peppers, carrots, broccoli, and other colorful vegetables contribute to an alkaline environment.
- **Fruits:** Berries, apples, pears, and citrus fruits are alkaline-forming and provide essential vitamins and minerals for hair health.
- **Nuts and Seeds:** Almonds, walnuts, flaxseeds, and chia seeds are alkaline and rich in healthy fats, protein, and nutrients.
- **Plant-Based Proteins:** Legumes (beans, lentils, peas), quinoa, and tofu are alkaline and provide protein for hair growth.

8. Reduced Acid-Forming Foods:

- **Animal Products:** Meat, dairy, and eggs are considered acid-forming and are limited on the alkaline diet.
- **Processed Foods:** Processed and refined foods, including sugary snacks and fast food, are generally acid-forming.

Tips for Incorporating the Alkaline Diet for Healthy Hair:

1. Focus on Fresh Produce:

- Aim to fill half your plate with a variety of colorful fruits and vegetables in every meal.

2. Choose Whole Grains:

- Opt for whole grains like quinoa, brown rice, and whole wheat, which are less acid-forming than refined grains.

3. Include Plant-Based Proteins:

- Incorporate plant-based protein sources such as beans, lentils, tofu, and tempeh into your meals.

4. Embrace Healthy Fats:

- Consume sources of healthy fats like avocados, nuts, seeds, and olive oil to support scalp health and hair shine.

5. Limit Processed Foods:

- Minimize processed and packaged foods that often contain added sugars, unhealthy fats, and additives.

6. Hydration is Key:

- Stay hydrated by drinking plenty of water and consuming water-rich foods like cucumbers, watermelon, and citrus fruits.

7. Plan Balanced Meals:

- Build well-balanced meals that include a combination of carbohydrates, protein, healthy fats, and a variety of nutrients.

8. Mindful Snacking:

- Choose alkaline snacks such as fresh fruits, raw vegetables with hummus, and nuts instead of processed snacks.

9. Experiment with Herbs and Spices:

- Use herbs and spices like turmeric, ginger, and basil to enhance flavor and provide additional health benefits.

10. Gradual Transition:

- If you're new to the alkaline diet, consider making gradual changes to your eating habits to allow your body to adjust.

11. Monitor Nutrient Intake:

- Ensure you're getting a balanced intake of nutrients, including protein, iron, zinc, and essential fatty acids, to support healthy hair growth.

12. Individualized Approach:

- Remember that everyone's nutritional needs are different. Consider working with a registered dietitian to tailor the alkaline diet to your specific health goals and requirements.

13. Be Patient:

- Changes in hair health take time. Consistently following a balanced diet and incorporating other healthy habits will contribute to long-term improvements.

14. Complement with Hair Care:

- Alongside dietary changes, maintain good hair care practices, including gentle handling, proper washing, and avoiding excessive heat styling.

Hair Care Practices for Preventing Hair Loss

Maintaining healthy hair requires a combination of good hair care practices, a balanced diet, and overall wellness. While certain hair loss factors are beyond your control, adopting a proper hair care routine can contribute to the health and strength of your hair. Here are detailed hair care practices to help prevent hair loss:

1. Gentle Hair Handling:

- **Avoid Tight Hairstyles:** Hairstyles that pull on the hair, such as tight ponytails and braids, can lead to hair breakage and stress on the hair follicles.

- **Use Soft Hair Accessories:** Choose hair ties, clips, and accessories that don't cause friction or breakage.

2. Proper Washing Technique:

- **Use Mild Shampoo:** Use a sulfate-free, mild shampoo that doesn't strip the hair of its natural oils.
- **Massage Gently:** While shampooing, use your fingertips to massage your scalp gently to improve blood circulation.
- **Rinse Thoroughly:** Make sure to rinse your hair thoroughly to remove all traces of shampoo and conditioner.

3. Scalp Health:

- **Keep Scalp Clean:** A clean scalp promotes healthy hair growth. Avoid excessive oil buildup, which can clog hair follicles.
- **Regular Cleansing:** Depending on your hair type, wash your hair as often as necessary to maintain scalp cleanliness.

4. Proper Conditioning:

- **Use Conditioner:** Apply a suitable conditioner to the lengths of your hair to prevent dryness and promote manageability.
- **Avoid Over-Conditioning:** Avoid applying conditioner to the scalp, as it can lead to excess oil buildup.

5. Heat Styling Precautions:

- **Heat Protection:** Always use a heat protectant spray before using hot styling tools to prevent damage.
- **Avoid Excessive Heat:** Limit the use of hair dryers, curling irons, and straighteners, as excessive heat can weaken hair and lead to breakage.

6. Nutrient-Rich Hair Treatments:

- **Hair Masks:** Apply natural hair masks with ingredients like coconut oil, avocado, and egg for added moisture and nutrients.

- **Scalp Massage:** Regular scalp massages with oils like coconut or jojoba can improve blood circulation to the hair follicles.

7. Proper Brushing and Combing:

- **Use Wide-Tooth Comb:** Start by detangling with a wide-tooth comb to prevent unnecessary hair breakage.
- **Gentle Brushing:** Use a soft-bristle brush or a detangling brush to brush your hair gently, starting from the ends and working your way up.

8. Avoid Over-Manipulation:

- **Avoid Over-Brushing:** Excessive brushing can lead to mechanical damage, especially when hair is wet.
- **Minimize Hair Pulling:** Refrain from twirling, twisting, or pulling on your hair, as it can weaken the strands.

9. Balanced Diet and Hydration:

- **Nutrient-Rich Diet:** Consume a balanced diet rich in vitamins, minerals, and proteins to support hair health.
- **Stay Hydrated:** Drink enough water to keep your body and hair well-hydrated.

10. Stress Management:

- **Stress Reduction:** Practice stress-reduction techniques such as meditation, yoga, or deep breathing to prevent stress-related hair loss.

11. Regular Trims:

- **Trim Split Ends:** Regular trims help prevent split ends from traveling up the hair shaft, maintaining hair health.

12. Avoid Harsh Chemicals:

- **Limit Hair Treatments:** Minimize the use of harsh chemical treatments like perms, relaxers, and bleaching, as they can weaken hair.

13. Choose Hair Products Wisely:

- **Use Sulfate-Free Shampoo:** Sulfates can strip natural oils from the hair and scalp, leading to dryness and irritation.
- **Check Ingredients:** Look for hair care products that are free from harsh chemicals and contain nourishing ingredients like natural oils and plant extracts.

14. Protect Hair from the Sun:

- **Wear a Hat:** When spending time outdoors, protect your hair and scalp from the sun's harmful UV rays by wearing a hat or using a scarf.
- **Use UV Protection:** Some hair care products contain UV protection to shield hair from sun damage.

15. Avoid Over-Washing:

- **Balance Washing Frequency:** Washing your hair too often can strip it of its natural oils. Find a balance that suits your hair type and lifestyle.

16. Choose Silk Pillowcases:

- **Gentler on Hair:** Silk or satin pillowcases create less friction than cotton, reducing hair breakage and friction.

17. Hair Extensions and Styles:

- **Choose Extensions Carefully:** If using hair extensions, opt for ones that are not too heavy or tight, which can stress the hair follicles.
- **Rotate Hairstyles:** Avoid wearing the same tight hairstyle regularly to prevent constant stress on the same areas of the scalp.

18. Know When to Seek Help:

- **Consult a Professional:** If you're experiencing excessive hair loss, changes in hair texture, or persistent scalp issues, consult a dermatologist or healthcare provider for proper evaluation and guidance.

19. Be Patient:

- **Hair Growth Takes Time:** Hair growth occurs gradually, and it may take several months to notice significant improvements. Be patient and consistent with your hair care routine.

20. Individualized Approach:

- **Tailor to Your Needs:** What works for one person may not work for another. Customize your hair care routine based on your hair type, concerns, and lifestyle.

Embracing Natural Beauty: Empowering Hair Care Choices

Embracing natural beauty in your hair care routine involves celebrating your unique hair texture, color, and pattern while making conscious choices that promote its health and vitality. This approach encourages self-confidence and empowers you to make informed decisions about your hair care practices. Here's a detailed exploration of how embracing natural beauty can lead to empowered hair care choices:

1. Understanding Hair Diversity:

- **Hair Texture:** Recognize that hair comes in various textures, from straight to wavy, curly, and coily. Embrace your natural texture rather than trying to conform to a certain standard.
- **Hair Color:** Whether your hair is naturally dark, light, or somewhere in between, appreciate its unique hue and avoid harsh chemical treatments that may damage it.

2. Nurturing Your Natural Hair:

- **Healthy Hair Practices:** Prioritize practices that promote hair health, such as gentle handling, proper washing, and using nourishing products.
- **Embrace Your Curls or Waves:** If you have curly or wavy hair, learn about techniques and products that enhance your natural pattern, reducing the need for heat styling.

3. Transitioning from Heat Styling:

- **Reducing Heat Usage:** Embrace heat-free hairstyles that showcase your hair's natural texture and reduce heat damage.
- **Protective Styles:** Experiment with protective hairstyles like braids, twists, and buns that shield your hair from excessive manipulation and external factors.

4. Avoiding Harmful Chemicals:

- **Minimize Chemical Treatments:** Limit or avoid harsh treatments like relaxers, perms, and excessive bleaching that can weaken and damage hair.
- **Natural Hair Dyes:** If you choose to color your hair, consider using natural hair dyes that are gentler on your hair and scalp.

5. Embracing Hair Growth Journey:

- **Patience:** Understand that hair growth is a gradual process. Embrace your hair growth journey and celebrate small milestones along the way.
- **Regular Trims:** Trim split ends regularly to maintain the health and strength of your hair as it grows.

6. Self-Expression and Confidence:

- **Own Your Unique Style:** Embrace the hairstyles that make you feel confident and authentic, whether it's a sleek ponytail, natural curls, or a bold color.
- **Inner Confidence:** True empowerment comes from feeling comfortable in your natural skin and knowing that your hair doesn't define your worth.

7. Education and Resources:

- **Learn About Your Hair:** Understand your hair's needs, porosity, and optimal care routines through educational resources, books, videos, and online communities.

8. Supportive Hair Care Products:

- **Curly Hair Care Products:** Explore hair care lines designed for your specific hair texture, which often include products formulated to enhance natural curls.
- **Gentle Ingredients:** Choose products with nourishing ingredients that enhance hair

health without causing damage.

9. Mindful Hair Styling:

- **Braids and Twists:** Experiment with protective styles like braids and twists that not only protect your hair but also offer versatility and creativity.
- **Accessories:** Use hair accessories like headbands, scarves, and hairpins to add flair to your natural hairstyles.

10. Self-Love and Acceptance:

- **Celebrating Diversity:** Recognize that beauty comes in all forms, and embracing your natural hair contributes to a more inclusive definition of beauty.

11. Self-Care Routine:

- **Relaxation:** Incorporate relaxation techniques into your hair care routine, such as scalp massages or aromatherapy, to make the experience more enjoyable.
- **Quality Time:** Dedicate time to care for your hair, treating it as a form of self-care and self-expression.

12. Embracing Changes:

- **Seasonal Changes:** Embrace how your hair might change with the seasons and adjust your routine accordingly.
- **Age and Life Changes:** Understand that hair may change over time due to factors like age, hormones, and lifestyle, and adapt your care routine accordingly.

13. Resisting Societal Pressures:

- **Challenge Norms:** Challenge societal beauty standards by proudly wearing your hair as you naturally intended, whether it's curly, coily, wavy, or straight.

Book 8: Cancer-Free Living: Dr. Sebi's Approach to Fighting Cancer Holistically

Understanding Cancer: Causes and Risk Factors

Cancer is a complex group of diseases characterized by the uncontrolled growth and spread of abnormal cells in the body. It can affect various organs and tissues and is a leading cause of morbidity and mortality worldwide. Understanding the causes and risk factors of cancer is crucial for prevention, early detection, and effective management. Here's a detailed explanation of the causes and risk factors associated with cancer:

1. Genetic Mutations:

- **Somatic Mutations:** Most cancers are caused by genetic mutations that occur in the DNA of cells during a person's lifetime. These mutations can disrupt the normal control mechanisms that regulate cell growth, division, and repair.
- **Inherited Mutations:** In some cases, individuals inherit genetic mutations from their parents that increase their risk of developing certain types of cancer, such as breast and ovarian cancer (BRCA mutations).

2. Carcinogens and Environmental Factors:

- **Chemical Carcinogens:** Exposure to certain chemicals and substances, such as tobacco smoke, asbestos, benzene, and formaldehyde, can increase the risk of cancer by damaging DNA and promoting the growth of abnormal cells.
- **Radiation Exposure:** Ionizing radiation from sources like excessive sun exposure, medical imaging tests (X-rays, CT scans), and radioactive substances can increase the risk of cancer by damaging DNA.

3. Lifestyle Factors:

- **Tobacco Use:** Smoking and exposure to secondhand smoke are major risk factors for several types of cancer, including lung, throat, mouth, and bladder cancer.
- **Diet:** A diet high in processed meats, red meats, sugary foods, and low in fruits and vegetables can contribute to an increased risk of various cancers.
- **Alcohol Consumption:** Heavy and regular alcohol consumption is associated with an elevated risk of cancers of the mouth, throat, esophagus, liver, breast, and more.

- **Physical Inactivity:** Lack of regular physical activity is linked to an increased risk of certain cancers.

4. Infections:

- **Viral Infections:** Some viruses, such as human papillomavirus (HPV), hepatitis B and C viruses, and Epstein-Barr virus, can lead to chronic infections that increase the risk of specific cancers.
- **Bacterial Infections:** H. pylori infection of the stomach lining is linked to an increased risk of stomach cancer.

5. Hormones:

- **Hormone Replacement Therapy (HRT):** Long-term use of hormone replacement therapy, particularly estrogen and progesterone after menopause, can increase the risk of breast and uterine cancer.

6. Family History and Genetic Predisposition:

- **Inherited Gene Mutations:** Genetic mutations that increase cancer risk can be passed down from parents to children, leading to a higher likelihood of developing certain cancers.

7. Age:

- **Increased Risk with Age:** The risk of developing cancer generally increases with age, as DNA mutations accumulate over time.

8. Gender and Hormonal Factors:

- **Gender:** Some cancers are more common in one gender than the other due to hormonal differences. For example, breast cancer is more prevalent in women, while prostate cancer is more common in men.

9. Ethnicity and Geographic Location:

- **Ethnicity:** Certain cancers are more prevalent in specific ethnic groups due to genetic, environmental, and lifestyle factors.

- **Geographic Location:** Environmental factors, such as exposure to specific carcinogens, can vary by region and contribute to varying cancer rates.

10. Occupational Exposures:

- **Workplace Carcinogens:** Certain occupations expose individuals to carcinogens, such as asbestos, arsenic, and benzene, increasing the risk of specific cancers.

11. Obesity:

- **Cancer Risk:** Obesity is linked to an increased risk of several types of cancer, including breast, colorectal, pancreatic, and kidney cancer.

12. Immune System Suppression:

- **Immunosuppression:** Individuals with weakened immune systems, such as those with HIV/AIDS or undergoing organ transplantation, are at a higher risk of certain cancers, including Kaposi sarcoma and lymphomas.

13. Chronic Inflammation:

- **Inflammatory Conditions:** Chronic inflammation caused by conditions like inflammatory bowel disease (Crohn's disease, ulcerative colitis) increases the risk of colorectal cancer.

14. Hormonal Factors:

- **Early Menstruation and Late Menopause:** Women who start menstruating at an early age or experience menopause at a late age are at a slightly higher risk of breast cancer due to prolonged exposure to estrogen.

15. Hormone Replacement Therapy (HRT):

- **Breast and Ovarian Cancer:** Long-term use of certain types of hormone replacement therapy (estrogen and progesterone) can increase the risk of breast and ovarian cancer.

16. Genetic Syndromes:

- **Hereditary Syndromes:** Genetic conditions like Lynch syndrome and familial adenomatous polyposis (FAP) increase the risk of colorectal and other cancers.

17. Personal Medical History:

- **Previous Cancer Diagnosis:** Individuals who have had cancer once are at a slightly higher risk of developing a second primary cancer.

18. Exposure to Hormones:

- **Oral Contraceptives:** Use of oral contraceptives may slightly increase the risk of certain cancers, such as breast and cervical cancer.

19. Preventive Measures:

- **Screening:** Regular screenings for specific cancers, such as mammograms for breast cancer and colonoscopies for colorectal cancer, can aid in early detection and treatment.
- **Vaccinations:** Vaccines like HPV vaccine and hepatitis B vaccine can prevent infections that are associated with increased cancer risk.

20. Comprehensive Approach:

- **Combined Risk Factors:** Many cancers result from the interplay of multiple risk factors, including genetic predisposition, lifestyle choices, and environmental exposures.

21. Individualized Risk Assessment:

- **Consult Healthcare Provider:** For individuals concerned about cancer risk, consulting with a healthcare provider can help assess personal risk factors and develop a tailored preventive plan.

Dr. Sebi's Herbal Support for Cancer Patients

Dr. Sebi, whose full name was Alfredo Darrington Bowman, was a self-proclaimed herbalist and natural healer. He advocated for an alkaline diet and the use of herbal remedies as a means to promote health and well-being. It's important to note that Dr. Sebi's approach and recommendations are not widely accepted by the mainstream medical community, and there is limited scientific evidence to support his claims. However, for the sake of explanation, here's an overview of some of the herbal recommendations Dr. Sebi reportedly made for cancer patients:

1. Sea Moss (Irish Moss):

- **Usage:** Dr. Sebi often recommended sea moss, a type of algae rich in nutrients, as a potential remedy to support overall health.

2. Bladderwrack:

- **Usage:** Bladderwrack, another type of seaweed, is believed to be rich in minerals and iodine and might have been suggested for its potential benefits.

3. Elderberry:

- **Usage:** Elderberry is often touted for its immune-boosting properties. Some proponents believe it may aid in promoting overall health.

4. Burdock Root:

- **Usage:** Burdock root is commonly used in herbal medicine and is believed to have detoxifying and blood-purifying properties.

5. Dandelion Root:

- **Usage:** Dandelion root is thought to have diuretic properties and may be used to support kidney health and detoxification.

6. Sarsaparilla:

- **Usage:** Sarsaparilla is traditionally used as a tonic and is believed by some to have potential health benefits.

7. Nutritional Guidelines:

- **Alkaline Diet:** Dr. Sebi advocated for an alkaline diet rich in plant-based foods, including fruits, vegetables, nuts, seeds, and whole grains. He believed that maintaining an alkaline pH in the body could support overall health.

Important Considerations:

- **Lack of Scientific Evidence:** Dr. Sebi's herbal recommendations and dietary guidelines lack robust scientific evidence supporting their efficacy in treating cancer or other health conditions.
- **Consult a Healthcare Provider:** Cancer is a serious medical condition that requires evidence-based medical treatment. It's essential for individuals diagnosed with cancer to consult qualified healthcare professionals, such as oncologists and medical doctors, for appropriate diagnosis and treatment plans.
- **Holistic Approach:** While some herbs may have potential health benefits, they should not be considered a substitute for proven medical interventions such as chemotherapy, radiation, surgery, and other evidence-based treatments for cancer.
- **Individualized Care:** Cancer treatment and management should be tailored to each individual's specific medical condition, needs, and preferences. Qualified medical professionals can provide personalized guidance.

Additional Considerations for Cancer Patients Seeking Herbal Support:

1. Complementary Approaches:

- **Integration with Medical Treatment:** If considering herbal remedies, it's important to communicate openly with your healthcare team to ensure that any herbal supplements or dietary changes do not interfere with your medical treatment plan.
- **Evidence-Based Care:** Rely on evidence-based medical interventions as the foundation of your cancer treatment plan, and view herbal remedies as potential complementary options.

2. Expert Guidance:

- **Consult a Healthcare Professional:** Before incorporating any herbal remedies into your routine, consult with your oncologist or healthcare provider to discuss potential interactions, risks, and benefits.
- **Qualified Herbalists:** If seeking herbal support, consider consulting a qualified herbalist or naturopath who has experience working with cancer patients and can provide personalized guidance.

3. Be Informed:

- **Research Carefully:** Before trying any herbal remedy, conduct thorough research and critically evaluate the available information. Look for reputable sources and studies.
- **Safety Concerns:** Keep in mind that some herbs can interact with medications, cause allergic reactions, or have side effects. Be cautious and informed.

4. Listen to Your Body:

- **Monitor Your Body:** Pay close attention to how your body responds to any herbal remedies. If you experience any adverse reactions, discontinue use and consult a healthcare professional.

5. Mind-Body Connection:

- **Stress Management:** Incorporating stress-reduction techniques, such as meditation, yoga, and deep breathing, can support your overall well-being during cancer treatment.

6. Nutritional Support:

- **Registered Dietitian:** Consult a registered dietitian with experience in oncology to create a balanced and nourishing diet that supports your health during cancer treatment.

7. Supportive Care:

- **Holistic Approach:** Embrace a holistic approach to cancer care that includes medical treatment, supportive care, and lifestyle practices that promote well-being.

8. Community Support:

- **Support Groups:** Joining cancer support groups or online communities can provide you with valuable insights, shared experiences, and emotional support.

9. Empowerment and Informed Choices:

- **Taking Control:** Empower yourself by staying informed about your treatment options and making informed choices that align with your values and preferences.

The Alkaline Diet for Cancer Management

The alkaline diet is a dietary approach that focuses on consuming foods that are believed to promote an alkaline pH in the body, aiming to support overall health and potentially impact conditions like cancer. The idea behind the alkaline diet is that acidic environments in the body might contribute to disease, including cancer, and that consuming alkaline-promoting foods can counteract this acidity. It's important to note that while the alkaline diet has gained popularity, scientific evidence supporting its efficacy in cancer management is limited. Here's a detailed exploration of the alkaline diet and its potential role in cancer management:

Key Principles of the Alkaline Diet:

- **Alkaline-Promoting Foods:** The diet emphasizes consuming foods that are considered alkaline-forming, such as fruits, vegetables, nuts, seeds, legumes, and some whole grains.
- **Acidic Foods to Limit:** The diet encourages reducing the intake of acidic foods, such as processed meats, refined sugars, dairy products, and some grains.

Potential Mechanism:

- **pH Balance:** Proponents of the alkaline diet suggest that by promoting a more alkaline pH in the body, it might create an environment less conducive to cancer growth. However, the body has natural mechanisms to regulate its pH levels, making it unlikely that diet alone significantly impacts overall pH.

The Alkaline Diet in Depth

Underlying Theory: The alkaline diet is grounded in the idea that the foods we eat can impact the body's pH level, influencing our health. The pH scale measures how acidic or alkaline a substance is, ranging from 0 (most acidic) to 14 (most alkaline). While different parts of the human body have varying pH levels, the blood's pH is tightly regulated around 7.35-7.45, slightly alkaline. The diet suggests that by consuming foods that are alkaline-forming in the body, one can potentially create a less hospitable environment for diseases like cancer.

Food Choices:

1. **Vegetables**: Cruciferous vegetables like broccoli, cauliflower, and Brussels sprouts are promoted for their anticancer properties. Other alkaline vegetables include kale, spinach, Swiss chard, beet greens, and cucumber.

2. **Fruits**: Most fruits are considered alkaline-forming. Berries, especially blueberries and raspberries, have been studied for their potential anticancer properties. Other alkaline fruits include melons, bananas, cherries, and grapes.

3. **Nuts and Seeds**: Almonds and chia seeds are particularly emphasized in the alkaline diet. They provide healthy fats and are considered less acid-forming compared to other nuts and seeds.

4. **Grains**: While many grains are slightly acidic, a few, like millet, amaranth, and quinoa, are more alkaline-forming.

5. **Legumes**: Lentils, chickpeas, and mung beans are examples of legumes that are more alkaline compared to others.

6. **Herbs and Spices**: Many herbs and spices are alkaline-forming, and they can also have additional health benefits. For instance, turmeric contains curcumin, which has been studied for its potential anticancer properties.

Foods to Limit or Avoid:

1. **Meats and Processed Meats**: These are typically acid-forming.

2. **Dairy Products**: Most dairy products are acidic.

3. **Processed Foods**: These often contain preservatives, artificial flavors, and other chemicals, making them highly acidic.

4. **Sugary Drinks and Snacks**: Excess sugar can lead to acidity.

5. **Excessive Caffeine and Alcohol**: Both can create an acidic environment when consumed in large amounts.

Water: Hydration is crucial in the alkaline diet. Alkaline water, which is ionized to increase its pH, is sometimes recommended, though its benefits over regular water are still debated.

Theoretical Benefits:

- **Detoxification**: By eliminating acidic foods and toxins from the diet, the body can potentially detoxify, improving overall health.

- **Improved Energy**: Some proponents report increased energy levels, possibly due to the higher intake of vitamins and minerals from plant-based foods.

- **Cancer Resistance**: The central claim is that cancer cells thrive in an acidic environment, and by making the body more alkaline, one might reduce the risk or hinder the progression of cancer.

Holistic Lifestyle Strategies for Cancer Prevention

Holistic Lifestyle Strategies for Cancer Prevention and the Alkaline Diet Approach

The journey to cancer prevention is multifaceted. While genetics plays a role, our daily choices significantly impact our health. Beyond mere dietary guidelines, a holistic approach to cancer prevention encapsulates mind, body, and environment. Within this broader perspective, the Alkaline Diet stands as a distinctive dietary approach. Let's examine how these strategies integrate for comprehensive cancer prevention.

1. Nutritional Choices: The Alkaline Diet:

- **Foundation**: The premise is that acid-forming foods can create an internal environment conducive to disease, including cancer. Conversely, alkaline-forming foods may help prevent disease.

- **Emphasis on Plant-Based Foods**: Fresh fruits, vegetables, nuts, seeds, and specific grains form the backbone of the diet. Not only are these foods alkaline-forming, but they also come packed with antioxidants, vitamins, and minerals, all of which play roles in cancer prevention.

- **Reduction of Acidic Foods**: Processed foods, meats, dairy, and excessive caffeine are minimized or eliminated due to their acidifying nature.

2. Mental and Emotional Well-being:

- **Stress Management**: Chronic stress can lead to inflammation, a precursor to many diseases, including cancer. Techniques such as meditation, deep breathing exercises, and yoga can alleviate stress.

- **Positive Relationships**: Building strong, positive relationships and fostering community can act as protective factors against many health conditions.

3. Physical Activity:

- **Regular Exercise**: Physical activity is directly linked to a reduced risk of certain cancers. It's essential for lymphatic drainage, boosting immunity, and reducing inflammation.

- **Connection with Nature**: Activities like hiking, gardening, or simply walking outdoors can connect us with our environment, providing both physical and mental health benefits.

4. Environmental Considerations:

- **Reducing Toxin Exposure**: This includes being mindful of the chemicals in our cleaning products, personal care items, and even the food we consume. Opting for organic produce, for instance, can reduce exposure to pesticides.

- **Mindful Consumption**: This pertains to both food and material goods, aiming for sustainability and reduced waste, which positively impacts overall environmental health.

5. Spiritual Connection:

- **Finding Purpose**: A sense of purpose or connection to something greater than oneself can offer solace, reduce stress, and provide clarity in life choices.

- **Practices**: Whether it's through organized religion, personal spiritual practices, or merely moments of reflection and gratitude, connecting with one's spiritual side can be a source of strength and resilience.

6. Continuous Learning and Adaptation:

- **Stay Updated**: Research and understanding about health and wellness continuously evolve. It's crucial to stay informed about the latest findings and adapt accordingly.

- **Personalized Approach**: Everyone's body is unique. Regular health check-ups, listening to one's body, and adjusting based on its needs is a holistic strategy in itself.

Thriving Beyond Cancer: Embracing a Life of Healing

Surviving cancer is a remarkable achievement, but the journey doesn't end with treatment completion. Thriving beyond cancer involves embracing a life of healing, growth, and renewed purpose. Here's a detailed exploration of how individuals can thrive after cancer:

1. Embracing Survivorship:

- **Acknowledge Accomplishments:** Celebrate your journey and the strength you've shown throughout the challenges.
- **Positive Mindset:** Cultivate a positive outlook on life, focusing on gratitude and the possibilities that lie ahead.

2. Physical Wellness:

- **Regular Health Check-ups:** Continue with regular medical appointments and screenings to monitor your health and catch any potential issues early.
- **Healthy Lifestyle:** Maintain a balanced diet, engage in regular exercise, and prioritize sleep to support overall physical well-being.

3. Emotional Well-being:

- **Address Emotions:** Understand that emotional healing is an ongoing process. Seek therapy, support groups, or counseling to address any lingering emotional challenges.
- **Mindfulness Practices:** Incorporate mindfulness, meditation, and relaxation techniques to manage stress and anxiety.

4. Setting Goals:

- **New Endeavors:** Set meaningful goals for your post-cancer life, whether they involve hobbies, career aspirations, or personal growth.

- **Dream Big:** Use your experience as motivation to pursue dreams and aspirations that bring fulfillment and happiness.

5. Reconnecting with Others:

- **Support Network:** Nurture your relationships with loved ones who supported you during your cancer journey.
- **New Connections:** Explore opportunities to connect with fellow survivors who understand your experiences.

6. Engaging in Meaningful Activities:

- **Passions and Hobbies:** Engage in activities that bring joy, purpose, and a sense of accomplishment.
- **Volunteer Work:** Contribute to your community or a cause close to your heart to foster a sense of fulfillment.

7. Gratitude and Mindfulness:

- **Gratitude Practice:** Cultivate a practice of gratitude to focus on the positives in your life and appreciate each moment.
- **Living Mindfully:** Embrace mindfulness to stay present and fully engage in daily activities.

8. Seeking Professional Support:

- **Therapy and Counseling:** If needed, continue therapy or counseling to address any psychological or emotional challenges.
- **Reintegration:** Work with therapists to navigate the transition back to daily life after treatment.

9. New Perspectives:

- **Renewed Outlook:** Use your experience to gain a new perspective on life's challenges and setbacks.
- **Personal Growth:** Embrace personal growth and self-discovery as you navigate the post-cancer journey.

10. Advocacy and Awareness:

- **Raise Awareness:** Use your story to raise awareness about cancer prevention, early detection, and survivorship.
- **Support Others:** Offer support to individuals currently going through the cancer journey, providing insights and encouragement.

11. Patience and Self-Compassion:

- **Be Kind to Yourself:** Understand that healing takes time, and it's okay to experience a range of emotions.
- **Self-Care:** Prioritize self-care to nurture your physical, emotional, and mental well-being.

12. Redefining Identity:

- **Beyond Cancer:** Explore your identity beyond being a cancer survivor. Define yourself by your interests, passions, and aspirations.

13. Self-Discovery:

- **Explore Passions:** Take the time to explore new interests and hobbies that bring you joy and fulfillment.

14. Creative Expression:

- **Art and Writing:** Engage in creative activities like art, writing, music, or dance as a form of self-expression and healing.

15. Body Image and Self-Confidence:

- **Positive Self-Image:** Work on cultivating a positive body image and self-confidence as you adjust to changes brought about by treatment.
- **Supportive Clothing:** Invest in clothing that makes you feel comfortable and confident.

16. Open Communication:

- **Share Your Journey:** Openly share your experiences with close friends, family, or support groups. Sharing can be cathartic and help others going through similar experiences.

17. Resilience and Adaptability:

- **Adapting to Change:** Embrace the ability to adapt to life's challenges and changes, drawing strength from the resilience you've developed.

18. Gratitude Journaling:

- **Daily Practice:** Keep a gratitude journal to record moments of gratitude and positivity in your life.

19. Spiritual Well-Being:

- **Spiritual Practices:** Engage in spiritual practices that resonate with you, whether through prayer, meditation, or mindfulness.

20. Time Management:

- **Prioritize Well-Being:** Manage your time in a way that allows for self-care, relaxation, and activities that bring you joy.

21. Holistic Approach to Health:

- **Mind, Body, Spirit:** Recognize the interconnectedness of your physical, emotional, and spiritual well-being.

22. Celebrate Milestones:

- **Personal Achievements:** Celebrate both small and significant milestones as you continue to make progress on your healing journey.

23. Embracing Uncertainty:

- **Living in the Moment:** Focus on the present moment and embrace the uncertainty that comes with life after cancer.

24. Advocating for Yourself:

- **Medical Care:** Continue advocating for your health by communicating openly with healthcare professionals and addressing any concerns.

25. Gratitude for Support:

- **Express Appreciation:** Thank those who supported you during your cancer journey, letting them know how much their presence meant to you.

26. Patience and Adaptation:

- **Life Transitions:** Recognize that adjusting to post-cancer life is a gradual process that requires patience and adaptation.

Conclusion:

Thriving beyond cancer is a deeply personal and transformative journey. By engaging in self-discovery, fostering creativity, cultivating self-confidence, and maintaining a holistic approach to health, individuals can navigate the challenges of life after cancer with grace and resilience. Remember that healing is a continuous process, and each step you take towards embracing a life of healing is a testament to your strength and determination. By nurturing your physical, emotional, and spiritual well-being and pursuing activities that bring joy and fulfillment, you can build a life that is vibrant, purposeful, and rich with possibilities.

Book 9: Breaking Free from Kidney Stones: Dr. Sebi's Natural Kidney Stone Solutions

Kidney Stones: Causes and Symptoms

Kidney stones, also known as renal calculi, are solid deposits that form in the kidneys. They can vary in size and composition and can cause significant discomfort when they block the urinary tract. Understanding the causes and symptoms of kidney stones is essential for prevention, early detection, and management. Here's a detailed exploration of kidney stones' causes and symptoms:

1. Causes of Kidney Stones:

- **Mineral Imbalances:** Kidney stones often form due to an imbalance of minerals and salts in the urine. The most common types of kidney stones are calcium stones and uric acid stones.
- **Dehydration:** Insufficient fluid intake can lead to concentrated urine, which increases the risk of stone formation.
- **Dietary Factors:** Consuming foods high in oxalate (found in spinach, chocolate, nuts) or animal protein can contribute to stone formation.
- **Family History:** A genetic predisposition to kidney stones can increase the likelihood of developing them.
- **Certain Medical Conditions:** Conditions like hyperparathyroidism, gout, and urinary tract infections can contribute to stone formation.
- **Obesity:** Obesity and a high body mass index (BMI) are associated with an increased risk of kidney stones.

2. Symptoms of Kidney Stones:

- **Pain:** The hallmark symptom of kidney stones is severe pain, often described as one of the most intense pains a person can experience. The pain can radiate from the back to the groin.
- **Flank Pain:** Pain typically originates in the back or side (flank) and may move to the lower abdomen and groin as the stone travels through the urinary tract.
- **Hematuria:** Blood in the urine, known as hematuria, is a common symptom of kidney stones. Urine may appear pink, red, or brown.

- **Painful Urination:** Individuals with kidney stones may experience a burning sensation or pain while urinating.
- **Frequency and Urgency:** Kidney stones can cause an increased frequency of urination and a sense of urgency.
- **Nausea and Vomiting:** The pain associated with kidney stones can lead to feelings of nausea and vomiting.
- **Cloudy or Foul-Smelling Urine:** In some cases, the presence of kidney stones can lead to changes in urine color and odor.

3. Types of Kidney Stones:

- **Calcium Stones:** The most common type, these stones are made primarily of calcium oxalate or calcium phosphate.
- **Uric Acid Stones:** Formed from uric acid, these stones can develop in people with high levels of uric acid in their urine.
- **Struvite Stones:** Often associated with urinary tract infections, these stones can grow quickly and cause significant complications.
- **Cystine Stones:** A rare type of stone that forms due to a genetic disorder that causes excessive cystine in the urine.

4. Complications:

- **Obstruction:** Kidney stones can block the urinary tract, causing severe pain and potential damage to the kidneys.
- **Infections:** An obstruction caused by kidney stones can lead to urinary tract infections.
- **Hydronephrosis:** Blockage of the urinary tract can cause urine to back up into the kidneys, leading to swelling and potential kidney damage.

5. Diagnosis:

- **Medical Evaluation:** If you suspect kidney stones, consult a healthcare professional who may perform a physical examination and order tests.
- **Imaging Tests:** Imaging tests like ultrasound, CT scans, or X-rays can help visualize the presence and location of kidney stones.

- **Urine Analysis:** Urine tests can reveal the presence of minerals and compounds that contribute to stone formation.

6. Prevention Strategies:

- **Hydration:** Drinking plenty of water throughout the day helps dilute urine and reduce the risk of stone formation.
- **Dietary Changes:** Depending on the type of stone, dietary adjustments can help manage risk. For instance, reducing oxalate-rich foods or animal protein.
- **Moderation:** While limiting certain foods, avoid extreme dietary changes that can lead to nutrient imbalances.
- **Medication:** In some cases, your healthcare provider might prescribe medications to prevent stone formation, such as thiazide diuretics or allopurinol.

7. Treatment Options:

- **Small Stones:** Small stones often pass on their own through increased fluid intake. Pain management and close monitoring are important.
- **Larger Stones:** Larger stones may require medical intervention. Treatments include extracorporeal shock wave lithotripsy (ESWL), ureteroscopy, or surgical removal.

8. Lifestyle Modifications:

- **Hygiene:** Maintain proper hygiene to prevent urinary tract infections that can contribute to stone formation.
- **Regular Physical Activity:** Engaging in regular exercise supports overall health and helps manage weight, which can reduce the risk of stone formation.

9. Medical Follow-Up:

- **Regular Check-ups:** If you've had kidney stones, follow your healthcare provider's recommendations for regular check-ups to monitor your kidney health.

10. Individualized Approach:

- **Consultation with Healthcare Provider:** Work closely with a healthcare professional to develop a personalized plan that addresses your specific risk factors and medical history.

11. Importance of Education:

- **Understanding Your Condition:** Educate yourself about kidney stones, their causes, and prevention strategies to make informed decisions.

12. Support and Resources:

- **Support Groups:** Consider joining support groups for individuals with kidney stones to share experiences and gain insights.

Dr. Sebi's Herbal Remedies for Kidney Stones

Dr. Sebi, a natural healer and herbalist, proposed an approach to health and healing that emphasizes the consumption of nutrient-rich, plant-based foods and herbs to support the body's natural healing processes. While there is limited scientific research on the effectiveness of Dr. Sebi's herbal remedies for kidney stones, his recommendations are rooted in promoting overall wellness. Here's an exploration of some of Dr. Sebi's herbal remedies that may be suggested for kidney stone management:

1. Dandelion Root:

- **Properties:** Dandelion root is believed to have diuretic properties, potentially aiding in increasing urine production and flushing out toxins.
- **Potential Benefit:** Increased urine production can help prevent the concentration of minerals and salts that contribute to kidney stone formation.

2. Uva Ursi:

- **Properties:** Uva ursi, also known as bearberry, is believed to have antimicrobial properties that may support urinary tract health.
- **Potential Benefit:** Supporting urinary tract health can be important in preventing urinary tract infections that can contribute to kidney stone formation.

3. Hydrangea Root:

- **Properties:** Hydrangea root is thought to have diuretic and anti-inflammatory properties.
- **Potential Benefit:** Diuretic properties may help increase urine flow, assisting in flushing out minerals that can lead to stone formation.

4. Corn Silk:

- **Properties:** Corn silk is believed to have diuretic properties and contains compounds that may support kidney health.
- **Potential Benefit:** Diuretic effects may aid in maintaining healthy urine flow, potentially reducing the risk of mineral buildup.

5. Chanca Piedra:

- **Properties:** Also known as "stone breaker," chanca piedra is believed to have potential diuretic and anti-inflammatory properties.
- **Potential Benefit:** It may help break down and prevent the formation of stones in the kidneys and urinary tract.

6. Nettle Leaf:

- **Properties:** Nettle leaf is rich in vitamins and minerals and is believed to have diuretic properties.
- **Potential Benefit:** Supporting healthy kidney function and increasing urine output can be beneficial in preventing stone formation.

7. Marshmallow Root:

- **Properties:** Marshmallow root is thought to have soothing and anti-inflammatory properties.
- **Potential Benefit:** It may help soothe urinary tract tissues and promote overall urinary tract health.

8. Buchu Leaf:

- **Properties:** Buchu leaf is believed to have potential diuretic and anti-inflammatory properties.

- **Potential Benefit:** It may contribute to increased urine flow and support urinary tract health.
- **Important Considerations:**
- **Individual Responses:** Herbal remedies can vary in effectiveness for different individuals. What works for one person may not work the same way for another.
- **Medical Guidance:** Before incorporating herbal remedies into your routine, consult a healthcare professional, especially if you have existing medical conditions, are taking medications, or are pregnant.
- **Holistic Approach:** Herbal remedies should be part of a comprehensive approach to kidney stone management, including hydration, dietary adjustments, and medical supervision.

9. Quality and Sourcing:

- **Choose Reputable Sources:** When using herbal remedies, ensure that you source them from reputable suppliers to ensure quality and authenticity.
- **Fresh vs. Dried Herbs:** Some herbs may be more potent when used fresh, while others are effective in dried form. Research the recommended form for each herb.

10. Dosage and Preparation:

- **Follow Guidelines:** Adhere to recommended dosages and preparation methods for each herbal remedy. Avoid excessive consumption, as it may lead to adverse effects.
- **Consultation with Herbalists:** Consider consulting with experienced herbalists who can provide personalized guidance on dosages and combinations of herbs.

11. Hydration and Dietary Adjustments:

- **Water Intake:** Continue to prioritize hydration, as sufficient fluid intake helps prevent mineral accumulation and supports overall kidney health.
- **Dietary Choices:** Dr. Sebi's approach to nutrition emphasizes plant-based, nutrient-rich foods. Incorporate a variety of fruits, vegetables, whole grains, and legumes.

12. Monitoring and Professional Guidance:

- **Healthcare Provider's Input:** Inform your healthcare provider about any herbal remedies you plan to use, especially if you have existing health conditions or are taking medications.
- **Monitoring Results:** Regularly monitor how your body responds to herbal remedies, and adjust your approach based on any changes you observe.

13. Lifestyle Factors:

- **Hygiene Practices:** Maintain good hygiene practices to prevent urinary tract infections, which can contribute to kidney stone formation.
- **Regular Physical Activity:** Engaging in regular physical activity can support overall health and contribute to kidney function.

14. Combined Approach:

- **Complementing with Medical Treatment:** Herbal remedies can complement medical treatment but should not replace it. Work in collaboration with your healthcare provider.

15. Patience and Consistency:

- **Time and Results:** Herbal remedies often require consistent use over time to potentially yield positive effects. Be patient and committed to the process.

The Alkaline Diet for Kidney Stone Prevention

The alkaline diet is based on the idea that consuming alkaline-forming foods can help maintain a slightly alkaline pH in the body, promoting overall health and preventing conditions like kidney stones. While scientific evidence on the direct impact of the alkaline diet on kidney stone prevention is limited, it emphasizes nutrient-rich, plant-based foods that align with principles of balanced nutrition. Here's a detailed exploration of the alkaline diet for kidney stone prevention:

1. Acid-Base Balance:

- **Understanding pH:** The pH scale measures acidity (below 7) and alkalinity (above 7). The alkaline diet aims to promote a more alkaline environment in the body.
- **Kidney Stone Connection:** An alkaline environment may help prevent the formation of certain types of kidney stones, such as calcium oxalate stones.

2. Alkaline-Forming Foods:

- **Fruits:** Most fruits, including berries, melons, citrus fruits, and avocados, are considered alkaline-forming.
- **Vegetables:** Many vegetables, such as leafy greens, broccoli, cauliflower, and bell peppers, are alkaline-forming.
- **Nuts and Seeds:** Almonds, chia seeds, flaxseeds, and walnuts are examples of alkaline-forming nuts and seeds.
- **Legumes:** Beans, lentils, and peas are alkaline-forming legumes.

3. Hydration:

- **Water's Alkaline Effect:** Drinking alkaline water may have a slight impact on maintaining alkalinity in the body.
- **Hydration's Role:** Staying well-hydrated is crucial for preventing kidney stone formation by maintaining proper urine volume and dilution.

4. Limiting Acid-Forming Foods:

- **Processed Foods:** Highly processed foods, sugary snacks, and sodas tend to be acid-forming.

- **Animal Proteins:** Meat, poultry, and dairy products are often considered acid-forming in the body.
- **Salt and Sodium:** Excessive salt intake can contribute to acid formation and disrupt calcium balance.

5. Calcium and Oxalate Balance:

- **Dietary Calcium:** Consuming adequate calcium from plant-based sources can bind to oxalate in the gut, reducing its absorption and risk of stone formation.
- **Oxalate-Rich Foods:** While some high-oxalate foods (spinach, rhubarb) are nutrient-rich, moderation is key to prevent excess oxalate intake.

6. Fiber-Rich Diet:

- **Whole Grains:** Incorporate whole grains like quinoa, brown rice, and oats for fiber, which supports digestive health.
- **Fruits and Vegetables:** High-fiber plant foods aid digestion and promote a healthy gut environment.

7. Plant-Based Proteins:

- **Legumes:** Beans, lentils, and chickpeas are excellent sources of plant-based protein.
- **Nuts and Seeds:** Almonds, chia seeds, and hemp seeds provide protein along with healthy fats.

8. Moderation and Balance:

- **Variety:** Embrace a variety of alkaline-forming foods to ensure a well-rounded nutrient intake.
- **Balanced Approach:** Balance the alkaline diet with other dietary principles, such as portion control and nutrient diversity.

9. Individualized Approach:

- **Health Needs:** Customize your alkaline diet based on your health status, preferences, and any underlying medical conditions.

10. Collaboration with Healthcare Professionals:

- **Medical Guidance:** Consult with healthcare professionals before making significant dietary changes, especially if you have kidney conditions or other health issues.

11. Portion Control:

- **Moderation:** While many alkaline-forming foods are healthy, portion control is important to prevent overconsumption of any nutrient.

12. Mindful Eating:

- **Slow and Mindful:** Practice mindful eating by eating slowly, savoring flavors, and paying attention to hunger and fullness cues.

13. Adequate Nutrient Intake:

- **Variety:** Ensure a diverse range of nutrient-rich foods to meet your body's nutritional needs.
- **Vitamin D:** Adequate vitamin D intake, often associated with sunlight exposure, is important for calcium absorption.

14. Combining with Other Strategies:

- **Hydration and Physical Activity:** Combine the alkaline diet with adequate hydration and regular physical activity for holistic kidney stone prevention.

15. Monitoring and Adjustment:

- **Personalized Approach:** Monitor your body's response to dietary changes and make adjustments as needed to find what works best for you.

16. Long-Term Lifestyle:

- **Sustainability:** Aim for a sustainable, long-term approach to the alkaline diet, considering its impact on overall health.

17. Consultation with Registered Dietitian:

- **Professional Guidance:** Consider consulting a registered dietitian who can provide personalized guidance based on your health status, dietary preferences, and goals.

Embracing Kidney Health: Empowering a Stone-Free Life

The kidneys, often overshadowed by the heart and brain, play a vital role in ensuring our body's smooth operation. Acting as natural filtration units, they cleanse the blood of toxins, help regulate blood pressure, and play a role in red blood cell production. Yet, when kidney stones form, they can wreak havoc on this smooth operation, causing immense pain and potential complications. To embrace kidney health is to empower ourselves with a life free from the clutches of these stones.

Understanding the genesis of kidney stones is the first step. These stones form when certain minerals and salts crystallize in the kidneys, often due to concentrated urine. Factors such as diet, hydration levels, genetics, and certain medical conditions can influence their formation.

Hydration is the cornerstone of kidney health. Drinking ample water ensures that our urine remains diluted, making it harder for crystals to form. The golden rule for most individuals is to aim for pale yellow urine, a sign of proper hydration. Moreover, water helps flush out toxins and smaller crystals before they conglomerate into bigger, problematic stones.

Dietary choices also play a pivotal role. Consuming a diet rich in oxalates, found in foods like spinach, rhubarb, and almonds, can increase the risk of calcium oxalate stones. On the other hand, high salt intake can elevate calcium in urine, leading to stone formation. To counteract this, incorporating a balanced diet with the right mix of minerals, salts, and hydration is key. This includes consuming adequate calcium from dietary sources, as calcium binds with oxalate in the gut, reducing its passage into the kidneys.

The influence of genetics cannot be ignored. Individuals with a family history of kidney stones are often more susceptible, making awareness and preventive measures even more critical for them.

Certain medical conditions, such as urinary tract infections, renal tubular acidosis, and certain metabolic disorders, can amplify the risk. Therefore, regular health check-ups and early detection of such conditions can act as a preventive shield.

But beyond these factors, embracing a lifestyle conducive to kidney health has broader implications. Limiting alcohol and caffeine, maintaining a healthy weight, and avoiding smoking are general wellness principles that indirectly benefit kidney health.

Creating a stone-free life is also about education and advocacy. Awareness campaigns, community workshops, and regular medical check-ups can ensure early detection and prevention.

In essence, our kidneys, those silent workhorses, deserve as much attention and care as any other organ. By understanding their function and the factors that jeopardize them, we can craft a life that not only keeps kidney stones at bay but also promotes overall well-being. Embracing kidney health is not merely a reactive step to prevent a painful condition but a proactive approach to holistic health and vitality.

Book 10: Heart Health Unleashed: Dr. Sebi's Guide to a Healthy Heart

Heart Disease: Risk Factors and Prevention

Heart disease, also known as cardiovascular disease, is a broad term encompassing various conditions that affect the heart and blood vessels. It is a leading cause of death worldwide, and understanding its risk factors and preventive measures is crucial for maintaining heart health. In this chapter, we'll delve into the details of heart disease risk factors and strategies for prevention:

1. Understanding Heart Disease:

- **Cardiovascular System:** The cardiovascular system includes the heart and blood vessels, responsible for circulating oxygen-rich blood throughout the body.
- **Types of Heart Disease:** Heart disease encompasses conditions such as coronary artery disease (CAD), heart attacks, heart failure, arrhythmias, and more.

2. Risk Factors for Heart Disease:

Modifiable Risk Factors:

- **Smoking:** Tobacco use damages blood vessels, increases blood pressure, and accelerates the development of atherosclerosis (artery narrowing).
- **Unhealthy Diet:** A diet high in saturated fats, trans fats, sodium, and added sugars contributes to obesity, high cholesterol, and high blood pressure.
- **Physical Inactivity:** Lack of regular exercise increases the risk of obesity, diabetes, high blood pressure, and overall cardiovascular risk.
- **Obesity:** Excess body weight strains the heart, raises blood pressure, and increases the likelihood of developing diabetes and high cholesterol.
- **High Blood Pressure:** Hypertension damages blood vessels, leading to atherosclerosis and heart strain.
- **High Cholesterol:** Elevated levels of "bad" LDL cholesterol contribute to plaque buildup in arteries.
- **Diabetes:** Diabetes affects blood vessel health and increases the risk of heart disease.
- **Stress:** Chronic stress may contribute to unhealthy lifestyle habits and strain on the heart.

Non-Modifiable Risk Factors:

- **Age:** As people age, the risk of heart disease increases.
- **Gender:** Men are generally at higher risk, but the risk for women increases after menopause.
- **Family History:** A family history of heart disease raises the risk.
- **Race and Ethnicity:** Some racial and ethnic groups are at higher risk.

3. Prevention Strategies:

Healthy Lifestyle Choices:

- **Balanced Diet:** Consume a diet rich in fruits, vegetables, whole grains, lean proteins, and healthy fats. Limit processed foods, sugary beverages, and excessive salt.
- **Regular Exercise:** Engage in at least 150 minutes of moderate-intensity aerobic activity or 75 minutes of vigorous-intensity activity per week.
- **Tobacco Cessation:** Quit smoking and avoid exposure to secondhand smoke.
- **Moderate Alcohol Intake:** If consuming alcohol, do so in moderation. Avoid excessive drinking.

Blood Pressure and Cholesterol Management:

- **Regular Check-ups:** Monitor blood pressure and cholesterol levels regularly.
- **Medication Adherence:** If prescribed, take medications for blood pressure and cholesterol as directed by healthcare professionals.
- **Stress Reduction:**
- **Stress Management:** Practice relaxation techniques, mindfulness, yoga, or meditation to manage stress.

Maintaining a Healthy Weight:

- **Caloric Balance:** Consume the appropriate number of calories for your activity level to maintain a healthy weight.

Regular Medical Check-ups:

- **Screening Tests:** Regular health screenings help detect and manage risk factors like blood pressure, cholesterol, and diabetes.

Education and Awareness:

- **Understanding Risk:** Educate yourself about heart disease risk factors, signs, and symptoms to make informed decisions.

4. Collaboration with Healthcare Professionals:

- **Medical Guidance:** Consult healthcare professionals for personalized recommendations based on your risk factors, medical history, and lifestyle.

5. Importance of Early Detection:

- **Screening:** Early detection and management of risk factors contribute to the prevention of heart disease.

6. Blood Sugar Management:

- **Diabetes Control:** If you have diabetes, work closely with your healthcare team to manage blood sugar levels through medication, diet, and lifestyle changes.

7. Sleep Quality:

- **Adequate Sleep:** Aim for 7-9 hours of quality sleep each night to support overall health and reduce cardiovascular risk.

8. Medication Management:

- **Adherence:** If prescribed medications for conditions like high blood pressure or cholesterol, take them consistently as directed by your healthcare provider.

9. Family Support:

- **Encourage Health:** Involve family members in adopting healthy lifestyle changes, creating a supportive environment for heart health.

10. Limiting Salt Intake:

- **Sodium Moderation:** Reduce sodium intake to help control blood pressure. Read food labels and choose low-sodium options.

11. Mindful Eating:

- **Portion Control:** Practice mindful eating by paying attention to portion sizes and eating slowly to recognize feelings of fullness.

12. Regular Health Assessments:

- **Routine Check-ups:** Schedule regular appointments with healthcare providers to assess your heart health and address any concerns.

13. Emotional Well-being:

- **Mental Health:** Prioritize emotional well-being through stress management, social connections, and seeking professional help if needed.

14. Community Support:

- **Support Groups:** Consider joining heart disease support groups to connect with others on similar health journeys.

15. Education Campaigns:

- **Public Awareness:** Participate in heart health awareness campaigns to spread knowledge and encourage preventive actions in your community.

16. CPR and First Aid Training:

- **Emergency Preparedness:** Learn CPR and basic first aid skills to respond effectively in case of cardiac emergencies.

17. Environment and Workplace:

- **Healthy Work Environment:** Create a heart-healthy workplace by encouraging physical activity, providing healthy snacks, and promoting stress reduction.

18. Limiting Alcohol Intake:

- **Moderation:** If you consume alcohol, limit it to moderate amounts as excessive drinking can contribute to heart disease risk.

19. Personalized Approach:

- **Tailored Recommendations:** Work with healthcare professionals to develop a personalized heart disease prevention plan based on your individual risk factors.

20. Stay Informed:

- **Latest Research:** Keep up with evolving research and guidelines related to heart disease prevention to make well-informed choices.

21. Teach Heart Health to Others:

- **Education:** Share your knowledge of heart disease risk factors and preventive measures with family, friends, and the community.

22. Long-Term Commitment:

- **Consistency:** Embrace heart-healthy habits as a lifelong commitment, consistently making choices that promote cardiovascular wellness.

23. Personal Motivation:

- **Intrinsic Reasons:** Reflect on your personal motivations for preventing heart disease, which may include improving quality of life, longevity, or being there for loved ones.

24. Setting a Positive Example:

- **Inspiration:** Your commitment to heart health can inspire others to make positive changes for their well-being.

Dr. Sebi's Herbal Support for Heart Health

Dr. Sebi was a herbalist and natural healer known for his holistic approach to health and wellness. He believed in the power of natural herbs and foods to support and maintain overall well-being, including heart health. While it's important to note that scientific evidence for specific herbal remedies can vary, here's a detailed exploration of some of the herbs that Dr. Sebi recommended for supporting heart health:

1. Hawthorn Berry (Crataegus spp.):

- **Benefits:** Hawthorn berry is believed to support cardiovascular health by improving blood circulation, dilating blood vessels, and supporting healthy blood pressure levels.
- **Usage:** It can be consumed as a tea, tincture, or in powdered form.

2. Garlic (Allium sativum):

- **Benefits:** Garlic is thought to have anti-inflammatory and antioxidant properties that support heart health. It may help lower cholesterol levels and regulate blood pressure.
- **Usage:** Garlic can be added to cooking or consumed as a supplement.

3. Cayenne Pepper (Capsicum annuum):

- **Benefits:** Cayenne pepper contains capsaicin, which may support heart health by improving blood circulation, reducing inflammation, and promoting healthy blood pressure levels.
- **Usage:** It can be used in cooking, added to beverages, or taken as a supplement.

4. Ginger (Zingiber officinale):

- **Benefits:** Ginger has anti-inflammatory properties and may help improve blood circulation, lower cholesterol levels, and reduce oxidative stress.
- **Usage:** Ginger can be added to foods, used to make tea, or taken as a supplement.

5. Linden Flower (Tilia spp.):

- **Benefits:** Linden flower is believed to have calming properties and may help support cardiovascular health by reducing stress and promoting relaxation.

- **Usage:** It can be consumed as a tea.

6. Burdock Root (Arctium lappa):

- **Benefits:** Burdock root is thought to have diuretic properties that may support heart health by promoting fluid balance and aiding in detoxification.
- **Usage:** It can be consumed as a tea, tincture, or in powdered form.

7. Bladderwrack (Fucus vesiculosus):

- **Benefits:** Bladderwrack is believed to contain iodine and other minerals that may support thyroid function and overall metabolism, indirectly impacting heart health.
- **Usage:** It's available in supplement form.

8. Ginger (Zingiber officinale):

- **Benefits:** Ginger has anti-inflammatory properties and may help improve blood circulation, lower cholesterol levels, and reduce oxidative stress.
- **Usage:** Ginger can be added to foods, used to make tea, or taken as a supplement.

9. Burdock Root (Arctium lappa):

- **Benefits:** Burdock root is thought to have diuretic properties that may support heart health by promoting fluid balance and aiding in detoxification.
- **Usage:** It can be consumed as a tea, tincture, or in powdered form.

10. Bladderwrack (Fucus vesiculosus):

- **Benefits:** Bladderwrack is believed to contain iodine and other minerals that may support thyroid function and overall metabolism, indirectly impacting heart health.
- **Usage:** It's available in supplement form.

11. African Bird Pepper (Capsicum annuum):

- **Benefits:** African bird pepper is believed to have potential benefits for cardiovascular health by improving blood circulation and supporting healthy blood pressure levels.
- **Usage:** It can be added to foods or used as a seasoning.

12. Nettle (Urtica dioica):

- **Benefits:** Nettle is thought to have diuretic properties that may aid in fluid balance and promote heart health.
- **Usage:** It can be consumed as a tea or added to foods.

13. Chaparral (Larrea tridentata):

- **Benefits:** Chaparral is believed to have antioxidant properties that may support heart health by reducing oxidative stress.
- **Usage:** It's available in supplement form.

14. Milk Thistle (Silybum marianum):

- **Benefits:** Milk thistle is thought to have liver-protective properties that indirectly support heart health by promoting overall detoxification.
- **Usage:** Milk thistle is often consumed as a supplement.

15. Elderberry (Sambucus spp.):

- **Benefits:** Elderberry is believed to have antioxidant and anti-inflammatory properties that support immune health, which can indirectly impact heart health.
- **Usage:** Elderberry can be consumed as a tea or in supplement form.

16. Chickweed (Stellaria media):

- **Benefits:** Chickweed is believed to have diuretic properties that may support heart health by aiding in fluid balance.
- **Usage:** It can be consumed as a tea or added to foods.

17. Dandelion (Taraxacum officinale):

- **Benefits:** Dandelion is thought to have diuretic properties that promote fluid balance and support overall detoxification, potentially benefiting heart health.
- **Usage:** Dandelion can be consumed as a tea, tincture, or in powdered form.

18. Lemon Balm (Melissa officinalis):

- **Benefits:** Lemon balm is believed to have calming properties that support relaxation, potentially benefiting heart health by reducing stress.
- **Usage:** Lemon balm can be consumed as a tea or added to foods.

19. Sea Moss (Chondrus crispus):

- **Benefits:** Sea moss is thought to contain minerals and nutrients that may indirectly support heart health by promoting overall vitality and well-being.
- **Usage:** Sea moss can be consumed in various forms, including as a gel or supplement.

20. Herbal Interactions:

- **Consultation:** Before incorporating multiple herbs or supplements, consult a healthcare professional to ensure they don't interact with each other or with any medications you're taking.

21. Quality and Purity:

- **Trusted Sources:** Choose reputable sources for herbal products to ensure their purity, quality, and absence of contaminants.

22. Individual Response:

- **Observation:** Pay attention to how your body responds to herbal remedies, and discontinue use if you experience any adverse reactions.

23. Dosage and Duration:

- **Guidance:** Follow recommended dosage instructions for herbs and supplements, and avoid exceeding recommended limits.

24. Integrative Approach:

- **Comprehensive Wellness:** Herbal remedies are just one part of a holistic approach to heart health. Combine them with other lifestyle factors for maximum benefit.

25. Tailored Approach:

- **Personalized Plan:** Work with a healthcare professional to create a personalized approach that considers your medical history, current health status, and overall wellness goals.

26. Regular Check-ups:

- **Health Monitoring:** Continue regular medical check-ups to assess your heart health and monitor any changes.

27. Lifestyle Alignment:

- **Holistic Harmony:** Integrate herbal support into a lifestyle that also includes balanced nutrition, exercise, stress management, and proper medical care.

28. Patience and Consistency:

- **Gradual Progress:** Herbal remedies may take time to show effects. Be patient and consistent in your approach.

29. Transparency with Healthcare Providers:

- **Communication:** Keep your healthcare providers informed about any herbal remedies you're using to ensure they can provide comprehensive care.

30. Individual Preferences:

- **Personal Choice:** Consider your preferences and comfort levels when deciding which herbal remedies to incorporate.

31. Holistic Balance:

- **Wellness Synergy:** Embrace a well-rounded approach to health that includes physical, emotional, mental, and spiritual well-being.

32. Professional Guidance:

- **Holistic Practitioner:** Consider consulting with holistic health practitioners who can provide guidance on herbal support within the context of your overall health.

33. Research and Education:

- **Informed Choices:** Stay informed about the latest research on herbal remedies and their potential benefits for heart health.

34. Ethical Sourcing:

- **Sustainability:** Choose herbs and supplements from sources that prioritize ethical and sustainable harvesting practices.

35. Cultural Considerations:

- **Cultural Wisdom:** Some herbal recommendations may stem from cultural traditions. Respect and explore the cultural context of the herbs you're considering.

The Alkaline Diet for a Strong Heart

The alkaline diet is based on the concept that consuming foods that promote an alkaline pH balance in the body can have various health benefits, including supporting heart health. While scientific evidence on the specific impact of the alkaline diet on heart health is still evolving, proponents suggest that it may contribute to a strong heart by encouraging the consumption of nutrient-rich foods and reducing the intake of processed and acidic foods. Let's explore the alkaline diet's principles and its potential benefits for heart health in detail:

1. Understanding the Alkaline Diet:

- **Acid-Alkaline Balance:** The alkaline diet aims to maintain the body's pH level slightly more alkaline, as opposed to being too acidic. This is believed to support overall health and well-being.

2. Alkaline-Forming Foods:

- **Fruits and Vegetables:** A major component of the alkaline diet, these foods are rich in vitamins, minerals, antioxidants, and fiber. They contribute to an alkaline pH when metabolized.
- **Leafy Greens:** Spinach, kale, collard greens, and Swiss chard are particularly alkaline-promoting and are associated with various health benefits.
- **Nuts and Seeds:** Almonds, flaxseeds, chia seeds, and walnuts are often recommended as alkaline sources of healthy fats and protein.

3. Acidic Foods to Limit:

- **Processed Foods:** Highly processed and refined foods, which often contain added sugars, unhealthy fats, and artificial additives, are typically acidic in nature.
- **Meat and Dairy:** While these are part of a balanced diet, excessive consumption of red meat and full-fat dairy products can contribute to an acidic environment.
- **Refined Grains:** Refined grains like white bread, pasta, and pastries are acid-forming due to their lack of fiber and nutrients.

4. Potential Benefits for Heart Health:

- **Nutrient Density:** The alkaline diet encourages the consumption of nutrient-rich foods like fruits and vegetables, which provide vitamins, minerals, and antioxidants that may support heart health.
- **Reducing Processed Foods:** By limiting processed and unhealthy foods, the alkaline diet aligns with heart-healthy dietary recommendations.
- **Fiber Intake:** Many alkaline-forming foods are high in fiber, which can help lower cholesterol levels and support digestive health.
- **Reducing Sodium:** The emphasis on whole, unprocessed foods may lead to reduced sodium intake, which can contribute to lower blood pressure.

5. Hydration:

- **Water:** Drinking sufficient water is integral to the alkaline diet. Proper hydration supports overall bodily functions, including cardiovascular health.

6. Plant-Based Emphasis:

- **Plant-Centric Diet:** The alkaline diet's focus on plant-based foods can lead to increased intake of phytonutrients, fiber, and heart-protective compounds.

7. Individual Variability:

- **Personalized Approach:** The alkaline diet may not suit everyone's needs. Individual responses to different foods can vary, so adjustments may be necessary.

8. Balanced Nutrition:

- **Comprehensive Diet:** While the alkaline diet promotes specific foods, it's important to ensure a balanced intake of all essential nutrients.

9. Consultation with Healthcare Professionals:

- **Professional Guidance:** Before making significant dietary changes, consult healthcare professionals, especially if you have existing health conditions.

10. Long-Term Lifestyle:

- **Sustainability:** Consider the long-term sustainability of the alkaline diet to ensure that it becomes a lifelong healthy eating pattern.

11. Mindful Eating:

- **Conscious Choices:** Pay attention to portion sizes and listen to your body's hunger and fullness cues.

12. Combining with Other Strategies:

- **Comprehensive Approach:** Consider combining the alkaline diet with other heart-healthy strategies like regular exercise, stress management, and medical guidance.

13. Health Monitoring:

- **Regular Check-ups:** Continue routine medical check-ups to monitor heart health and overall well-being.

14. Personal Enjoyment:

- **Diverse Diet:** Embrace a variety of foods that support heart health while also bringing joy to your meals.

15. Balanced Macronutrients:

- **Adequate Protein:** Ensure that you're getting enough protein from plant-based sources to support muscle maintenance and overall health.

16. Variety and Diversity:

- **Nutrient Spectrum:** Include a wide variety of alkaline-forming foods to ensure you're getting a diverse range of nutrients.

17. Cooking Methods:

- **Healthy Preparation:** Opt for cooking methods that retain the nutritional integrity of foods, such as steaming, roasting, or sautéing.

18. Mindful Food Choices:

- **Listening to Your Body:** Pay attention to how different foods make you feel and adjust your diet accordingly.

19. Gradual Changes:

- **Transitioning:** If transitioning to the alkaline diet, make gradual changes to allow your body to adapt to new eating patterns.

20. Social and Cultural Considerations:

- **Contextual Awareness:** Consider how the alkaline diet aligns with your social and cultural preferences and obligations.

21. Hydration Importance:

- **Balanced Fluid Intake:** Adequate water consumption is key for overall health and complements the alkaline diet's principles.

22. Nutrient Supplementation:

- **Professional Advice:** If you're considering supplements to support specific nutrients, consult healthcare professionals for guidance.

23. Holistic Approach:

- **Comprehensive Wellness:** Combine the alkaline diet with other health-promoting practices like stress reduction, exercise, and sufficient sleep.

24. Educational Resources:

- **Evidence-Based Information:** Rely on credible sources for information about the alkaline diet's potential benefits and limitations.

25. Personal Goals:

- **Clear Intentions:** Define your specific health goals and assess how the alkaline diet aligns with them.

26. Family and Community Support:

- **Shared Values:** Engage your family and community in understanding and supporting your dietary choices.

27. Positive Mindset:

- **Optimistic Outlook:** Approach the alkaline diet with a positive attitude, embracing the potential benefits it can offer.

28. Self-Reflection:

- **Regular Assessment:** Periodically reflect on how the alkaline diet is affecting your health and well-being.

29. Feedback from Professionals:

- **Health Monitoring:** Regularly check in with healthcare professionals to assess any changes in your health status.

30. Lifelong Learning:

- **Evolving Knowledge:** Stay open to new research and information about the alkaline diet's impact on heart health.

31. Cultural Adaptations:

- **Cultural Integration:** Modify the alkaline diet to suit your cultural food preferences while still adhering to its core principles.

Exercise and Lifestyle for Cardiovascular Health

Regular physical activity and a heart-healthy lifestyle play pivotal roles in promoting cardiovascular health. Engaging in regular exercise, adopting a balanced diet, managing stress, getting adequate sleep, and avoiding harmful habits contribute to maintaining a strong and resilient heart. In this chapter, we'll delve into the importance of exercise and lifestyle factors for cardiovascular health:

1. Physical Activity and Cardiovascular Health:

- **Exercise Benefits:** Regular physical activity strengthens the heart muscle, improves blood circulation, reduces blood pressure, and enhances overall cardiovascular function.
- **Types of Exercise:** Incorporate aerobic exercises (e.g., walking, jogging, swimming) and strength training to ensure a comprehensive workout routine.
- **Frequency and Duration:** Aim for at least 150 minutes of moderate-intensity aerobic exercise or 75 minutes of vigorous-intensity exercise per week, along with muscle-strengthening activities.

2. Nutrition for Heart Health:

- **Balanced Diet:** Embrace a diet rich in fruits, vegetables, whole grains, lean proteins, and healthy fats.
- **Limit Saturated and Trans Fats:** Minimize the consumption of saturated and trans fats, which can contribute to elevated cholesterol levels.
- **Omega-3 Fatty Acids:** Include sources of omega-3 fatty acids, such as fatty fish (salmon, mackerel) and flaxseeds, which are beneficial for heart health.
- **Fiber-Rich Foods:** Consume foods high in soluble fiber (oats, beans, fruits, vegetables) to help lower cholesterol levels.
- **Sodium Moderation:** Limit sodium intake to support healthy blood pressure levels.

3. Stress Management:

- **Stress Reduction Techniques:** Practice relaxation methods such as meditation, deep breathing, yoga, and mindfulness to lower stress levels.

- **Physical Activity:** Exercise helps reduce stress hormones and promotes a sense of well-being.

4. Adequate Sleep:

- **Sleep Quality:** Aim for 7-9 hours of quality sleep each night to support overall cardiovascular health.
- **Sleep Apnea Awareness:** Address sleep apnea, a condition associated with increased cardiovascular risk, if you experience symptoms.

5. Avoiding Harmful Habits:

- **Smoking Cessation:** Quit smoking and avoid exposure to secondhand smoke, as smoking damages blood vessels and increases heart disease risk.
- **Limit Alcohol Intake:** If you consume alcohol, do so in moderation. Excessive drinking can raise blood pressure and contribute to heart issues.

6. Regular Health Check-ups:

- **Routine Assessments:** Regular medical check-ups help monitor blood pressure, cholesterol levels, and other cardiovascular risk factors.
- **Health Screenings:** Undergo recommended health screenings to detect and manage conditions like diabetes and high cholesterol.

7. Staying Hydrated:

- **Adequate Fluid Intake:** Drink plenty of water to maintain proper hydration, which supports overall cardiovascular function.

8. Social Connections:

- **Supportive Relationships:** Cultivate social connections and maintain positive relationships, as they contribute to emotional well-being and stress reduction.

9. Mindful Eating:

- **Conscious Consumption:** Practice mindful eating by savoring meals, listening to hunger cues, and avoiding overeating.

10. Regular Health Assessments:

- **Health Monitoring:** Periodically assess your cardiovascular health and make necessary adjustments to your exercise and lifestyle routine.

11. Personalized Approach:

- **Individualized Strategies:** Customize your exercise and lifestyle choices based on your preferences, needs, and health goals.

12. Consultation with Healthcare Professionals:

- **Medical Guidance:** Consult healthcare professionals before making significant lifestyle changes, especially if you have existing health conditions.

13. Positive Mindset:

- **Optimism:** Maintain a positive outlook, as a positive mindset can contribute to overall well-being and motivation.

14. Combining Strategies:

- **Holistic Approach:** Integrate regular exercise, balanced nutrition, stress management, and other lifestyle factors for optimal cardiovascular health.

15. Continual Learning:

- **Staying Informed:** Stay up-to-date with evolving research on cardiovascular health and wellness.

16. Warm-up and Cool-down:

- **Proper Preparation:** Prior to exercise, warm up to gradually increase heart rate and circulation. Afterward, cool down to gradually lower heart rate.

17. Progressive Approach:

- **Gradual Increase:** When starting an exercise routine, gradually increase intensity and duration to prevent injury.

18. Hydration during Exercise:

- **Fluid Balance:** Drink water before, during, and after exercise to stay adequately hydrated.

19. Incorporate Movement into Daily Life:

- **Active Lifestyle:** Incorporate physical activity into your daily routine, such as taking the stairs or walking during breaks.

20. Setting Realistic Goals:

- **Achievable Objectives:** Set achievable exercise and lifestyle goals that align with your fitness level and time availability.

21. Diverse Activities:

- **Variety:** Engage in a variety of physical activities to prevent boredom and work different muscle groups.

22. Group Activities:

- **Social Engagement:** Participate in group exercises or sports to enhance motivation and create a sense of community.

23. Seek Professional Guidance:

- **Fitness Experts:** Consult with fitness professionals or trainers to create a safe and effective exercise plan.

24. Exercise Modifications:

- **Adaptations:** Modify exercises if you have any pre-existing conditions or physical limitations.

25. Heart Rate Monitoring:

- **Pulse Check:** Monitor your heart rate during exercise to ensure you're working within your target range.

26. Listening to Your Body:

- **Body Awareness:** Pay attention to your body's signals and adjust your exercise intensity as needed.

27. Outdoor Activities:

- **Nature's Benefits:** Engaging in outdoor exercises can have additional benefits for mental well-being.

28. Time Management:

- **Prioritize Exercise:** Schedule regular exercise sessions in your daily routine to make them a consistent habit.

29. Positive Self-Talk:

- **Motivational Thoughts:** Maintain a positive self-dialogue to encourage adherence to your exercise and lifestyle goals.

30. Tracking Progress:

- **Journaling:** Keep a record of your exercise and lifestyle changes to track your progress and stay motivated.

31. Family Involvement:

- **Shared Goals:** Encourage family members to join you in adopting a heart-healthy lifestyle.

32. Social Support:

- **Motivational Network:** Share your goals with friends or online communities to receive encouragement and support.

33. Environmental Considerations:

- **Safe Conditions:** Choose safe environments for exercise, whether indoors or outdoors.

34. Consistency:

- **Sustainable Routine:** Consistency is key. Make exercise and heart-healthy habits an integral part of your daily life.

35. Embracing Enjoyment:

- **Fun Factor:** Choose physical activities you enjoy to make exercise a rewarding experience.

Book 11: Easing Arthritis: Dr. Sebi's Natural Remedies for Arthritis

Understanding Arthritis: Types and Symptoms

Arthritis is a complex group of diseases characterized by inflammation and pain in the joints. It affects millions of people worldwide and can have a significant impact on their quality of life. There are numerous types of arthritis, each with distinct causes, symptoms, and treatments. In this chapter, we will delve into the details of arthritis, including its various types and the symptoms associated with each:

Arthritis Overview:

Inflammation of Joints: Arthritis refers to the inflammation of one or more joints, leading to pain, stiffness, and reduced mobility.

Chronic Condition: Most types of arthritis are chronic, meaning they persist over time, potentially causing long-term joint damage.

Osteoarthritis (OA):

Degenerative Arthritis: OA is the most common type of arthritis, characterized by the breakdown of joint cartilage over time.

Symptoms: Joint pain, stiffness (especially in the morning), decreased range of motion, and joint swelling.

Risk Factors: Age, obesity, joint injuries, and genetic predisposition.

Rheumatoid Arthritis (RA):

Autoimmune Disorder: RA is an autoimmune condition where the immune system attacks the synovium, the lining of the joints.

Symptoms: Joint pain, swelling, morning stiffness, fatigue, and systemic symptoms like fever.

Risk Factors: Genetics, hormonal factors, and environmental triggers.

Psoriatic Arthritis (PsA):

Associated with Psoriasis: PsA occurs in individuals with psoriasis and affects both skin and joints.

Symptoms: Joint pain, swelling, skin patches, nail changes, and inflammation.

Ankylosing Spondylitis (AS):

Spinal Involvement: AS primarily affects the spine and sacroiliac joints, leading to inflammation and potential fusion.

Symptoms: Lower back pain, stiffness, limited mobility, and discomfort in the hips and shoulders.

Juvenile Idiopathic Arthritis (JIA):

Affects Children: JIA refers to arthritis that begins before the age of 16, with various subtypes and presentations.

Symptoms: Joint pain, swelling, stiffness, and potential impact on growth and development.

Gout:

Uric Acid Buildup: Gout is caused by the accumulation of uric acid crystals in the joints, leading to sudden, intense pain.

Symptoms: Severe joint pain, redness, swelling, and tenderness, often affecting the big toe.

Lupus Arthritis:

Linked to Lupus: Lupus is an autoimmune disease that can also affect the joints.

Symptoms: Joint pain, swelling, fatigue, skin rashes, and other systemic symptoms.

Other Types of Arthritis:

Inflammatory Arthritis: This category includes less common forms like reactive arthritis, enteropathic arthritis, and more.

Symptoms Shared by Many Types:

Pain: Joint pain is a common symptom, often worsened by movement and activity.

Stiffness: Stiffness in the joints, particularly after periods of rest or inactivity, is a hallmark of arthritis.

Swelling: Inflamed joints can become swollen and tender to the touch.

Limited Range of Motion: Reduced mobility and difficulty moving joints are often experienced.

Warmth and Redness: Inflammation can lead to warmth and redness around affected joints.

Diagnosis:

Physical Examination: Doctors assess joint appearance, swelling, and range of motion.

Imaging: X-rays, MRI, and ultrasound help visualize joint damage and inflammation.

Blood Tests: Elevated levels of certain markers can indicate inflammation.

Treatment Approaches:

Medications: Pain relievers, anti-inflammatory drugs, disease-modifying antirheumatic drugs (DMARDs), and biologics.

Physical Therapy: Exercises to improve joint function, strength, and flexibility.

Lifestyle Modifications: Weight management, joint protection techniques, and assistive devices.

Managing Arthritis:

Disease Management: Regular medical check-ups and adherence to treatment plans.

Pain Management: Utilizing pain relief strategies, both pharmaceutical and non-pharmaceutical.

Lifestyle Changes: Adopting a balanced diet, staying physically active, managing stress, and getting sufficient sleep.

Consultation with Healthcare Professionals:

Medical Guidance: Seek medical advice for proper diagnosis, treatment, and management of arthritis.

Support Networks:

Support Groups: Connect with others living with arthritis to share experiences and coping strategies.

Prevention and Early Intervention:

Risk Reduction: Address modifiable risk factors such as obesity, joint injuries, and certain lifestyle habits.

Early Treatment: Seek medical attention at the first signs of joint discomfort to prevent worsening of symptoms and potential joint damage.

Holistic Approach:

Comprehensive Care: Consider the impact of arthritis on emotional well-being, mental health, and overall quality of life.

Impact on Daily Life:

Functional Limitations: Recognize how arthritis can affect daily activities, work, and hobbies.

Adapting Activities: Modify activities to accommodate joint discomfort and reduce strain.

Joint Protection:

Proper Techniques: Learn techniques to protect your joints during physical activities and everyday tasks.

Environmental Modifications:

Home Adaptations: Make adjustments at home to make daily tasks easier and reduce joint stress.

Pacing Activities:

Balanced Approach: Avoid overexertion by pacing yourself during physical activities and tasks.

Weather Sensitivity:

Climate Considerations: Some individuals with arthritis may experience changes in symptoms based on weather conditions.

Medication Management:

Medical Supervision: Work closely with healthcare professionals to monitor medication use and potential side effects.

Emotional Well-Being:

Psychological Impact: Acknowledge the emotional toll of arthritis and consider seeking support from mental health professionals if needed.

Family and Caregiver Support:

Educational Outreach: Ensure that family members and caregivers understand arthritis to provide adequate support.

Healthy Coping Strategies:

Stress Management: Engage in relaxation techniques, mindfulness, and hobbies to manage stress.

Open Communication:

Doctor-Patient Communication: Maintain open and honest communication with healthcare providers to ensure effective treatment and management.

Empowerment Through Education:

Informed Decisions: Understand your specific type of arthritis and available treatment options to make informed choices.

Long-Term Outlook:

Variable Course: The course of arthritis varies from person to person, so individual experiences may differ.

Promoting Awareness:

Public Education: Raise awareness about arthritis to reduce stigma and increase understanding.

Quality of Life Focus:

Holistic Health: Prioritize overall well-being and adjust your lifestyle to accommodate the challenges of arthritis.

Advocacy and Support:

Advocate for Yourself: Be an advocate for your health by actively participating in your treatment plan.

Incorporating Complementary Therapies:

Alternative Approaches: Some individuals explore complementary therapies like acupuncture, massage, or herbal supplements.

Exploring Assistive Devices:

Adaptive Tools: Consider using assistive devices to make daily tasks more manageable.

Future Research:

Advancements: Stay informed about the latest research and treatment options as medical knowledge continues to evolve.

Dr. Sebi's Herbal Recommendations for Arthritis

Dr. Sebi was a renowned holistic healer and herbalist who believed in using natural remedies to support various health conditions, including arthritis. His approach focused on alkaline foods and herbs that he believed could help restore balance in the body. Keep in mind that Dr. Sebi's recommendations are based on his own philosophies, and it's important to consult a healthcare professional before making any significant changes to your treatment plan. Here are some herbal recommendations commonly associated with Dr. Sebi's approach to managing arthritis:

1. Burdock Root:

- **Anti-inflammatory:** Burdock root is believed to possess anti-inflammatory properties that may help reduce joint pain and inflammation associated with arthritis.
- **Detoxification:** Dr. Sebi suggested that burdock root aids in detoxifying the body by promoting the elimination of waste and toxins.

2. Devil's Claw:

- **Pain Relief:** Devil's claw is thought to have analgesic and anti-inflammatory effects, potentially providing relief from arthritis-related pain.
- **Joint Health:** Dr. Sebi's approach suggests that devil's claw may contribute to maintaining joint health and flexibility.

3. Ginger:

- **Anti-Inflammatory:** Ginger is recognized for its anti-inflammatory properties, which could help alleviate arthritis symptoms.
- **Digestive Aid:** Dr. Sebi often emphasized the importance of good digestion, and ginger is believed to support healthy digestion.

4. Bromide Plus Powder:

- **Nutrient-Rich:** Dr. Sebi's Bromide Plus Powder is a blend of various herbs and sea moss, rich in essential nutrients that are believed to support overall health and well-being.
- **Alkaline Balance:** The blend is touted for its alkaline properties, which align with Dr.

Sebi's emphasis on maintaining an alkaline body pH.

5. Nettle:

- **Anti-Inflammatory:** Nettle is thought to possess anti-inflammatory qualities that could help alleviate joint pain and inflammation.
- **Nutrient Source:** Dr. Sebi's philosophy on nettle likely stems from its nutrient content, including vitamins, minerals, and antioxidants.

6. Chaparral:

- **Antioxidant Properties:** Chaparral is believed to contain antioxidants that may contribute to reducing oxidative stress associated with inflammation.
- **Cleansing:** Dr. Sebi's approach suggests that chaparral aids in the body's cleansing processes.

7. Sarsaparilla:

- **Anti-Inflammatory:** Sarsaparilla is thought to have anti-inflammatory properties that could offer relief from arthritis symptoms.
- **Detoxification:** Dr. Sebi's teachings emphasize the importance of detoxification, and sarsaparilla is believed to support this process.

8. Hydrangea Root:

- **Joint Health:** Hydrangea root is believed to promote joint health and mobility, potentially benefiting those with arthritis.
- **Anti-Inflammatory:** Dr. Sebi's recommendations likely stem from hydrangea root's purported anti-inflammatory effects.

9. Sea Moss:

- **Nutrient-Rich:** Sea moss is rich in essential minerals and nutrients that are believed to support overall health.
- **Alkaline Balance:** Dr. Sebi's approach emphasizes maintaining an alkaline body pH, and sea moss is considered alkaline.

10. Nopal:

- **Anti-Inflammatory:** Nopal, also known as prickly pear cactus, is believed to have anti-inflammatory properties that could help manage arthritis symptoms.
- **Digestive Health:** Dr. Sebi often stressed the importance of good digestion, and nopal is thought to support digestive health.

11. Plant-Based Diet:

- **Alkaline Foods:** Dr. Sebi's approach emphasizes an alkaline diet rich in fruits, vegetables, whole grains, and plant-based proteins.
- **Anti-Inflammatory Benefits:** Consuming a variety of plant-based foods may help reduce inflammation and support joint health.

12. Aloe Vera:

- **Anti-Inflammatory:** Aloe vera is believed to have anti-inflammatory properties that could contribute to alleviating arthritis symptoms.
- **Digestive Support:** Dr. Sebi's teachings often mention aloe vera for its potential to support digestion and nutrient absorption.

13. Dandelion Root:

- **Anti-Inflammatory:** Dandelion root is thought to possess anti-inflammatory effects that could benefit those with arthritis.
- **Liver Health:** Dr. Sebi's philosophy may stem from dandelion root's potential to support liver health and detoxification.

14. Yellow Dock Root:

- **Detoxification:** Yellow dock root is believed to support detoxification and elimination of waste from the body.
- **Potential Anti-Inflammatory:** Dr. Sebi's recommendations may be influenced by its potential anti-inflammatory effects.

15. Alfalfa:

- **Nutrient-Rich:** Alfalfa is rich in vitamins, minerals, and antioxidants, supporting overall health.
- **Alkaline Properties:** Dr. Sebi's approach aligns with the alkaline nature of alfalfa.

16. Copaiba:

- **Anti-Inflammatory:** Copaiba is believed to have anti-inflammatory properties that could offer relief from arthritis symptoms.
- **Pain Management:** Dr. Sebi's recommendations may be influenced by its potential analgesic effects.

17. Hemp Oil:

- **Anti-Inflammatory:** Hemp oil is recognized for its anti-inflammatory properties, potentially aiding in arthritis symptom management.
- **Nutrient Source:** Hemp oil is rich in essential fatty acids, which can support overall health.

18. Horsetail:

- **Joint Health:** Horsetail is thought to support joint health, potentially benefiting those with arthritis.
- **Silica Content:** Dr. Sebi's approach might consider horsetail's silica content, which is believed to contribute to connective tissue health.

19. Sage:

- **Antioxidant Properties:** Sage is believed to possess antioxidants that can help reduce oxidative stress associated with inflammation.
- **Cognitive Health:** Dr. Sebi's philosophy may align with sage's potential benefits for cognitive health.

20. White Willow Bark:

- **Natural Pain Relief:** White willow bark contains compounds similar to aspirin and is believed to provide natural pain relief.

- **Inflammation Reduction:** Dr. Sebi's approach might consider its potential to reduce inflammation and pain.

The Alkaline Diet for Arthritis Relief

The alkaline diet is a dietary approach that emphasizes consuming foods that have an alkalizing effect on the body, with the goal of maintaining a balanced pH level. While scientific evidence supporting the direct impact of the alkaline diet on arthritis is limited, some proponents believe that it may help alleviate symptoms by reducing inflammation and promoting overall health. Here's a detailed exploration of the alkaline diet and its potential benefits for arthritis relief:

1. Alkaline Diet Principles:

- **Alkaline vs. Acidic Foods:** The diet categorizes foods as either alkaline or acidic based on their potential impact on the body's pH level.
- **Balancing pH:** The alkaline diet aims to promote a slightly alkaline pH level in the body, which proponents believe supports optimal health.

2. Alkaline Diet Foods:

- **Alkaline-Rich Foods:** Fruits, vegetables, nuts, seeds, legumes, and whole grains are often considered alkaline-forming.
- **Acidic Foods:** Highly processed foods, animal products, caffeine, and alcohol are typically considered acidic-forming.

3. Potential Benefits for Arthritis:

- **Reducing Inflammation:** The alkaline diet emphasizes anti-inflammatory foods, which may contribute to alleviating arthritis-related inflammation and pain.
- **Nutrient Intake:** A diet rich in alkaline foods provides essential nutrients, antioxidants, and phytochemicals that support overall health and immune function.

4. Possible Mechanisms:

- **Balanced pH:** Proponents suggest that maintaining an alkaline pH can reduce the risk of chronic inflammation associated with certain types of arthritis.
- **Bone Health:** The diet's emphasis on fruits and vegetables might provide nutrients that support bone health, especially important in osteoarthritis.

5. Balanced Approach:

- **Variety and Moderation:** A balanced alkaline diet includes a variety of nutrient-dense foods and avoids extremes.
- **Individualized Approach:** Customizing the diet to personal preferences, allergies, and health needs is essential for long-term adherence.

6. Incorporating Alkaline Foods:

- **Leafy Greens:** Spinach, kale, and Swiss chard are nutrient-packed alkaline foods.
- **Colorful Vegetables:** Bell peppers, broccoli, carrots, and other colorful vegetables offer vitamins, minerals, and antioxidants.
- **Fruits:** Include alkaline fruits like berries, citrus fruits, and melons for their rich nutrient content.
- **Plant-Based Proteins:** Legumes, lentils, quinoa, and nuts provide plant-based protein while being alkaline-forming.
- **Healthy Fats:** Avocado, coconut, and certain nuts are sources of healthy fats that can be part of an alkaline diet.

7. Limiting Acidic Foods:

- **Processed Foods:** Highly processed foods often contain additives and preservatives and are usually considered acidic.
- **Animal Products:** Animal proteins, dairy, and eggs are generally acidic-forming in the body.
- **Sugar and Sweets:** Sugary foods and sweetened beverages are typically acidic and should be consumed in moderation.

8. Hydration and Alkalinity:

- **Water Quality:** Drinking alkaline water is promoted by some proponents, but research on its specific benefits for arthritis is limited.

9. Managing Portion Sizes:

- **Caloric Intake:** Pay attention to portion sizes to manage weight, which can impact arthritis symptoms, especially in weight-bearing joints.

10. Consultation with Healthcare Professionals:

- **Medical Guidance:** Before making significant dietary changes, consult a healthcare provider, especially if you have existing health conditions or take medications.

11. Potential Limitations:

- **Scientific Support:** While the alkaline diet has theoretical benefits, scientific evidence directly linking it to arthritis relief is lacking.
- **Individual Responses:** Responses to the diet may vary, and it might not offer significant relief for all individuals with arthritis.

12. Comprehensive Approach:

- **Combining Strategies:** The alkaline diet can be part of a holistic approach that includes medical treatment, exercise, stress management, and other lifestyle adjustments.

13. Balancing Macronutrients:

- **Protein Intake:** Choose plant-based protein sources, such as legumes, tofu, and quinoa, to support joint health and reduce potential inflammation.
- **Healthy Fats:** Include sources of healthy fats like avocados, nuts, seeds, and olive oil to provide essential fatty acids and support overall well-being.

14. Fiber-Rich Diet:

- **Digestive Health:** A diet rich in fiber from fruits, vegetables, and whole grains supports digestive health, which can indirectly impact inflammation and arthritis symptoms.

- **Satiety:** High-fiber foods contribute to feelings of fullness, potentially aiding in weight management.

15. Antioxidant-Rich Foods:

- **Colorful Produce:** Include a variety of colorful fruits and vegetables to benefit from their antioxidant content, which can help counteract oxidative stress.

16. Hydration:

- **Importance of Water:** Staying well-hydrated supports overall health and aids in the elimination of toxins.
- **Lemon Water:** Some proponents suggest starting the day with a glass of alkaline lemon water to support digestion and hydration.

17. Mindful Eating:

- **Slow and Enjoyable:** Practice mindful eating by savoring each bite, chewing thoroughly, and paying attention to hunger and fullness cues.

18. Adapting the Diet:

- **Personalized Approach:** Adjust the alkaline diet to meet individual preferences, cultural influences, and health needs.

19. Monitoring Progress:

- **Self-Reflection:** Keep a journal to track your diet, symptoms, and changes in arthritis-related discomfort.

20. Collaboration with Healthcare Professionals:

- **Medical Oversight:** Continue to work closely with healthcare providers to ensure a comprehensive approach to arthritis management.

21. Complementary Lifestyle Strategies:

- **Exercise:** Regular physical activity, tailored to your abilities, can support joint health, flexibility, and overall well-being.

- **Stress Management:** Engage in relaxation techniques like yoga, meditation, or deep breathing to reduce stress and its potential impact on arthritis symptoms.

22. Seeking Professional Guidance:

- **Registered Dietitian:** Consider consulting a registered dietitian with expertise in arthritis and nutrition to create a personalized eating plan.

23. Dietary Supplementation:

- **Supplement Use:** If considering supplements for arthritis relief, consult a healthcare professional to ensure they align with your specific needs and conditions.

24. Long-Term Lifestyle Approach:

- **Sustainability:** Aim for a balanced, sustainable approach to eating that supports your health and well-being over the long term.

25. Individual Responses:

- **Varied Results:** Responses to dietary changes can vary widely among individuals; what works for one person may not work for another.

Lifestyle Practices for Arthritis Management

Managing arthritis involves more than just dietary changes; it encompasses a holistic approach that considers various lifestyle practices. By adopting a comprehensive strategy, individuals with arthritis can optimize their well-being, reduce symptoms, and improve their overall quality of life. Here's a detailed exploration of lifestyle practices for arthritis management:

1. Regular Physical Activity:

- **Joint Health:** Engaging in low-impact exercises such as walking, swimming, and cycling helps maintain joint flexibility and reduce stiffness.
- **Muscle Strengthening:** Incorporating strength training helps support the muscles around joints, offering added stability and protection.
- **Range of Motion Exercises:** Gentle stretching and range of motion exercises maintain joint mobility and flexibility.

2. Weight Management:

- **Impact on Joints:** Maintaining a healthy weight reduces stress on weight-bearing joints like hips, knees, and ankles.
- **Inflammation:** Weight management can also help lower overall inflammation, which is beneficial for arthritis management.

3. Stress Management:

- **Mind-Body Techniques:** Practices like yoga, meditation, deep breathing, and mindfulness can help manage stress and reduce its impact on arthritis symptoms.
- **Coping Strategies:** Developing effective ways to cope with stressors enhances emotional well-being.

4. Quality Sleep:

- **Restorative Rest:** Adequate and high-quality sleep supports tissue repair and reduces inflammation, which can benefit arthritis management.
- **Sleep Hygiene:** Establish a sleep routine, create a comfortable sleep environment, and

avoid stimulants before bedtime.

5. Assistive Devices:

- **Mobility Aids:** Canes, walkers, and braces provide added support and stability, reducing stress on joints.
- **Ergonomic Tools:** Use ergonomic tools and adaptive devices to minimize joint strain during daily activities.

6. Joint Protection Techniques:

- **Body Mechanics:** Learn proper body mechanics to avoid joint strain during activities like lifting, bending, and carrying.
- **Adaptive Techniques:** Modify activities and use assistive devices to reduce joint stress.

7. Hot and Cold Therapy:

- **Pain Relief:** Applying heat or cold to affected joints can provide temporary relief from pain and stiffness.
- **Inflammation Management:** Cold therapy can help reduce inflammation, while heat therapy relaxes muscles and improves circulation.

8. Hydration:

- **Joint Lubrication:** Staying hydrated supports joint lubrication and can ease joint discomfort.

9. Ergonomic Environment:

- **Work and Home Setup:** Create ergonomic workstations and living spaces to minimize joint strain.

10. Social Support:

- **Emotional Well-Being:** Connecting with friends, family, and support groups fosters emotional well-being and reduces feelings of isolation.

11. Time Management:

- **Pacing Activities:** Break tasks into manageable segments to prevent overexertion and joint fatigue.

12. Medical Care:

- **Regular Check-Ups:** Maintain regular appointments with healthcare professionals to monitor arthritis progression and adjust treatment plans.
- **Medication Management:** Adhere to prescribed medications and discuss any concerns or side effects with your doctor.

13. Mindful Nutrition:

- **Balanced Diet:** Consume a well-rounded diet rich in fruits, vegetables, whole grains, and lean proteins to support overall health and inflammation reduction.
- **Hydration:** Ensure adequate fluid intake to support joint lubrication and overall well-being.

14. Moderate Alcohol and Tobacco Use:

- **Inflammation Reduction:** Limit alcohol consumption and avoid smoking, as both can contribute to inflammation and worsen arthritis symptoms.

15. Professional Support:

- **Registered Dietitian:** Consult a registered dietitian with expertise in arthritis to create a personalized eating plan.
- **Physical Therapist:** Seek guidance from a physical therapist to develop a tailored exercise program.

16. Adapting to Changes:

- **Flexibility:** Be open to adapting your lifestyle practices as your arthritis symptoms and needs evolve.

17. Positive Mindset:

- **Optimism:** Cultivate a positive outlook and focus on what you can do rather than what you can't.
- **Self-Compassion:** Be kind to yourself and acknowledge your efforts in managing arthritis.

18. Cognitive-Behavioral Strategies:

- **Pain Management:** Learn techniques to manage pain perception and reduce its impact on daily life.

19. Adaptive Strategies:

- **Energy Conservation:** Prioritize activities and plan breaks to prevent excessive fatigue and joint strain.
- **Task Simplification:** Break tasks into smaller steps to make them more manageable.

20. Physical Rest and Relaxation:

- **Balancing Activity and Rest:** Incorporate rest periods throughout the day to prevent overexertion.
- **Relaxation Techniques:** Practice deep breathing, progressive muscle relaxation, or guided imagery to reduce stress and tension.

21. Communication:

- **Open Dialogue:** Communicate your needs and limitations to friends, family, and colleagues, fostering understanding and support.

22. Environmental Modifications:

- **Accessibility:** Make your living space and workplace more accessible by removing obstacles and installing handrails if necessary.

23. Creative Outlets:

- **Hobbies:** Engage in creative activities that bring joy and relaxation, such as painting, music, or crafting.

24. Professional Support:

- **Occupational Therapist:** Consult an occupational therapist for guidance on adapting your environment and activities to your arthritis needs.
- **Psychologist or Counselor:** Seek emotional support and coping strategies from mental health professionals.

25. Personalized Approach:

- **Tailored Solutions:** Every individual's experience with arthritis is unique, so tailor your lifestyle practices to suit your specific needs.

26. Adapting Over Time:

- **Changing Needs:** As arthritis symptoms change, adapt your lifestyle practices to maintain their effectiveness.

27. Consistency:

- **Routine:** Establish consistent daily routines that include exercise, relaxation, and self-care.

28. Education and Empowerment:

- **Understanding:** Learn about arthritis, its symptoms, and treatment options to make informed decisions.
- **Self-Advocacy:** Advocate for your needs and rights in healthcare and everyday situations.

29. Social Engagement:

- **Support Networks:** Connect with others who have arthritis to share experiences, information, and emotional support.

30. Celebrating Progress:

- **Small Achievements:** Acknowledge and celebrate the progress you make in managing your arthritis.

31. Self-Care:

- **Balanced Lifestyle:** Prioritize self-care activities that bring you joy, relaxation, and well-being.

32. Holistic Health Focus:

- **Mind, Body, and Spirit:** Approach arthritis management holistically, considering physical, emotional, and spiritual well-being.

33. Planning for Flare-Ups:

- **Contingency Plans:** Have strategies in place to manage increased symptoms during flare-ups.

34. Patience:

- **Adapting to Changes:** Be patient with yourself as you navigate the ups and downs of living with arthritis.

Living Comfortably with Arthritis: Empowering a Pain-Free Life

Living comfortably with arthritis involves embracing a holistic approach that encompasses physical, emotional, and lifestyle considerations. By integrating various strategies and practices, individuals can empower themselves to lead a fulfilling life while minimizing pain and maximizing overall well-being. Here's a detailed exploration of how to live comfortably with arthritis and empower a pain-free life:

1. Holistic Self-Care:

- **Mind-Body Connection:** Recognize the interconnectedness of physical and emotional well-being in managing arthritis.
- **Self-Care Rituals:** Establish a routine of self-care practices that nurture both your body and mind.

2. Gentle Movement:

- **Low-Impact Activities:** Engage in exercises that promote joint health without putting excessive strain on affected areas.
- **Yoga and Tai Chi:** Gentle practices like yoga and tai chi improve flexibility, balance, and overall well-being.

3. Pain Management Techniques:

- **Mindful Pain Awareness:** Develop awareness of pain triggers and use relaxation techniques to manage discomfort.
- **Heat and Cold Therapy:** Apply heat or cold to affected joints to alleviate pain and reduce inflammation.

4. Adaptive Living:

- **Home Modifications:** Make necessary adjustments to your living space for improved accessibility and comfort.
- **Assistive Devices:** Use aids like ergonomic tools, braces, and mobility devices to support daily activities.

5. Positive Mindset:

- **Resilience:** Cultivate resilience and focus on your strengths to overcome challenges posed by arthritis.
- **Gratitude:** Practice gratitude to foster a positive outlook and shift your focus toward what you can enjoy.

6. Emotional Well-Being:

- **Stress Reduction:** Engage in stress-reduction techniques like meditation, deep breathing, and progressive muscle relaxation.
- **Support Systems:** Seek emotional support from friends, family, and support groups to navigate the emotional aspects of arthritis.

7. Nutrient-Rich Diet:

- **Inflammation Reduction:** Consume foods rich in antioxidants, omega-3 fatty acids, and anti-inflammatory compounds.
- **Hydration:** Stay well-hydrated to support joint lubrication and overall health.

8. Regular Medical Check-Ups:

- **Monitoring:** Maintain regular appointments with healthcare professionals to track arthritis progression and adjust treatment plans.
- **Medication Adherence:** Follow prescribed medications and communicate any concerns or side effects to your doctor.

9. Optimal Sleep:

- **Sleep Hygiene:** Create a comfortable sleep environment and practice good sleep hygiene to improve sleep quality.
- **Pain Management:** Adequate sleep supports pain management and overall well-being.

10. Creative Expression:

- **Artistic Outlets:** Engage in creative activities that bring joy, such as painting, writing, or playing a musical instrument.

11. Mindfulness Practices:

- **Present-Moment Awareness:** Practice mindfulness to stay grounded in the present and manage stress effectively.

12. Social Engagement:

- **Connections:** Cultivate relationships that offer emotional support, understanding, and companionship.

13. Education and Advocacy:

- **Informed Choices:** Learn about arthritis, treatment options, and self-care practices to make informed decisions.
- **Self-Advocacy:** Advocate for your needs in healthcare and daily life situations.

14. Empowerment:

- **Self-Efficacy:** Believe in your ability to manage arthritis and live a fulfilling life.
- **Taking Control:** Take an active role in your health, making choices that align with your well-being goals.

15. Celebrating Small Wins:

- **Personal Achievements:** Acknowledge and celebrate your progress, no matter how small.

16. Continued Learning:

- **Staying Informed:** Stay open to learning about new arthritis management strategies and advancements.

17. Balanced Approach:

- **Flexibility:** Adjust your lifestyle practices as needed while keeping a balanced perspective.

18. Setting Realistic Goals:

- **Achievable Objectives:** Set achievable goals for each day and celebrate your accomplishments.
- **Pacing Yourself:** Break larger tasks into smaller steps to avoid overexertion and fatigue.

19. Adaptive Socializing:

- **Social Activities:** Participate in social activities that align with your comfort level and energy.
- **Open Communication:** Communicate your needs to friends and family, ensuring they understand your limitations.

20. Professional Support:

- **Occupational Therapist:** Consult an occupational therapist for guidance on adapting your daily activities and environment.
- **Psychological Support:** Seek therapy to address emotional challenges and develop effective coping strategies.

21. Meaningful Engagement:

- **Purposeful Activities:** Engage in activities that bring a sense of purpose and fulfillment to your life.

22. Graded Exposure:

- **Gradual Challenges:** Gradually expose yourself to activities that you may have avoided due to arthritis-related concerns.

23. Mindful Movement:

- **Body Awareness:** Practice mindful movement to tune into your body's signals and prevent overexertion.

24. Journaling:

- **Reflection:** Keep a journal to reflect on your journey, track progress, and express your thoughts and emotions.

25. Advocacy and Support:

- **Community Engagement:** Connect with arthritis advocacy groups to stay informed and engage with others who share similar experiences.

26. Respect for Limits:

- **Listening to Your Body:** Pay attention to your body's signals and honor its limits to prevent pushing yourself too hard.

27. Resilience Building:

- **Problem-Solving Skills:** Develop problem-solving skills to effectively navigate challenges that arise due to arthritis.

28. Routine and Consistency:

- **Stability:** Establish a daily routine that includes self-care practices, exercise, rest, and relaxation.

29. Visualization Techniques:

- **Positive Imagery:** Use visualization to imagine yourself engaging in activities without pain or discomfort.

30. Engagement in Nature:

- **Nature's Calming Effect:** Spend time in nature to benefit from its calming and healing influence.

31. Holistic Support System:

- **Healthcare Team:** Collaborate with a team of healthcare professionals who specialize in arthritis care.
- **Personal Support:** Surround yourself with friends, family, and caregivers who understand and support your journey.

32. Sharing Your Experience:

- **Inspiration:** Share your experience with others to inspire and support those on a similar path.

33. Continuous Learning:

- **Adapting to Change:** Stay open to trying new strategies and approaches as your needs evolve over time.

34. Mindful Adaptation:

- **Flexible Approach:** Continuously adapt your lifestyle practices to changing circumstances and arthritis-related challenges.

Book 12: Clear Skin Naturally: Dr. Sebi's Approach to Radiant Skin

Skin Health: Common Skin Issues and Causes

Healthy skin plays a crucial role in our overall well-being, and understanding common skin issues and their underlying causes is essential for maintaining optimal skin health. This chapter will delve into various skin conditions, their causes, and factors that contribute to skin problems:

Acne:

Causes: Acne is often caused by excess oil production, clogged pores, bacteria, hormonal fluctuations, and inflammation.

Types: Different types of acne include whiteheads, blackheads, papules, pustules, nodules, and cysts.

Contributing Factors: Hormonal changes, genetics, diet, stress, and certain medications can contribute to acne.

Eczema (Atopic Dermatitis):

Causes: Eczema is a chronic skin condition characterized by inflamed, itchy, and dry skin. Genetics and immune system dysfunction play a role.

Triggers: Allergens, irritants, weather changes, stress, and certain foods can trigger eczema flare-ups.

Psoriasis:

Causes: Psoriasis is an autoimmune disorder where skin cells reproduce too quickly, leading to thick, red, scaly patches.

Immune System: Genetic predisposition and immune system abnormalities are primary causes.

Triggers: Infections, stress, injury, and some medications can trigger psoriasis episodes.

Rosacea:

Causes: Rosacea is characterized by facial redness, visible blood vessels, and often eye irritation. The exact cause is unknown.

Triggers: Factors like sunlight, alcohol, spicy foods, stress, and certain skincare products can trigger rosacea flare-ups.

Hives (Urticaria):

Causes: Hives are raised, itchy welts that appear suddenly. Allergies, stress, infections, and medications are common causes.

Histamine Release: Allergic reactions trigger the release of histamine, leading to hives.

Contact Dermatitis:

Causes: Contact dermatitis occurs when the skin reacts to an irritant (irritant contact dermatitis) or allergen (allergic contact dermatitis).

Irritants and Allergens: Common irritants include detergents and chemicals, while allergens can be metals, plants, or fragrances.

Skin Infections:

Causes: Bacterial, fungal, and viral infections can lead to skin issues like impetigo, ringworm, and warts.

Contagious: Some skin infections, like ringworm and warts, are contagious.

Skin Aging:

Causes: Skin aging is a natural process influenced by genetic factors, sun exposure, lifestyle, and collagen breakdown.

Sun Damage: UV radiation from the sun accelerates skin aging by breaking down collagen and elastin fibers.

Hyperpigmentation:

Causes: Hyperpigmentation results from an overproduction of melanin, often due to sun exposure, hormones, or inflammation.

Melasma: Hormonal changes, such as pregnancy or birth control use, can lead to melasma, a form of hyperpigmentation.

Dry Skin:

Causes: Dry skin occurs when the skin's natural barrier is compromised, leading to water loss and flakiness.

Environmental Factors: Cold weather, low humidity, and harsh skincare products can contribute to dry skin.

Skin Cancer:

Causes: Skin cancer is primarily caused by UV radiation from the sun or tanning beds damaging skin cells' DNA.

Risk Factors: Fair skin, history of sunburns, excessive sun exposure, and family history increase the risk.

Allergic Reactions:

Causes: Allergic reactions manifest as hives, redness, itching, or swelling due to the immune system's response to an allergen.

Common Allergens: Common allergens include certain foods, medications, insect stings, and latex.

Seborrheic Dermatitis:

Causes: Seborrheic dermatitis leads to scaly, red patches on the skin, often affecting the scalp (dandruff) and face.

Yeast Overgrowth: An overgrowth of a yeast called Malassezia on the skin is believed to contribute.

Vitiligo:

Causes: Vitiligo is an autoimmune disorder where the immune system attacks and destroys melanocytes, leading to depigmentation.

Genetic and Immune Factors: Genetics and immune system dysfunction are thought to play a role.

Warts:

Causes: Warts are caused by the human papillomavirus (HPV), leading to the formation of raised, rough growths on the skin.

Contagious: Warts can spread through skin-to-skin contact or by touching surfaces with the virus.

Dr. Sebi's Herbal Support for Healthy Skin

Dr. Sebi, also known as Alfredo Darrington Bowman, was a prominent herbalist and advocate for natural healing through plant-based diets and holistic approaches. He believed that the body could heal itself through proper nutrition and detoxification. Dr. Sebi's approach to herbal support for healthy skin centered around utilizing specific herbs that he believed could aid in promoting skin health and addressing various skin issues. Here are some of the herbs that Dr. Sebi commonly recommended for healthy skin and their potential benefits:

1. Burdock Root (Arctium lappa):

- **Benefits:** Burdock root is believed to have detoxifying properties, helping to cleanse the blood and promote healthy skin.
- **Anti-Inflammatory:** Its anti-inflammatory properties may aid in managing skin conditions like acne and eczema.

2. Yellow Dock (Rumex crispus):

- **Benefits:** Yellow dock is thought to support the liver and promote detoxification, which may indirectly contribute to clearer skin.
- **Blood Cleansing:** It's believed to assist in purifying the blood, which can have positive effects on skin health.

3. Sarsaparilla (Smilax spp.):

- **Benefits:** Sarsaparilla is often associated with skin health due to its potential blood-purifying properties.

- **Detoxification:** Its detoxifying effects are thought to help address skin conditions by eliminating toxins from the body.

4. Burdock Root (Arctium lappa):

- **Benefits:** Burdock root is believed to have detoxifying properties, helping to cleanse the blood and promote healthy skin.
- **Anti-Inflammatory:** Its anti-inflammatory properties may aid in managing skin conditions like acne and eczema.

5. Sea Moss (Chondrus crispus):

- **Benefits:** Sea moss is a type of seaweed rich in minerals and nutrients, which can support overall health and skin vitality.
- **Nutrient-Rich:** Sea moss contains vitamins, minerals, and antioxidants that may promote skin health and radiance.

6. Bladderwrack (Fucus vesiculosus):

- **Benefits:** Bladderwrack is another type of seaweed that contains minerals and compounds that may benefit skin health.
- **Iodine Content:** Its iodine content can support thyroid function, indirectly influencing skin health.

7. Dandelion (Taraxacum officinale):

- **Benefits:** Dandelion is believed to support liver function and detoxification, which can impact skin health.
- **Liver Health:** A healthy liver contributes to clearer skin by eliminating toxins and promoting proper digestion.

8. Bromide Plus Powder:

- **Benefits:** Dr. Sebi's Bromide Plus Powder is a blend of sea moss and bladderwrack, rich in minerals that can benefit overall health, including skin.
- **Mineral Support:** The minerals in this powder can nourish the body and potentially improve skin health.

9. Elderberry (Sambucus nigra):

- **Benefits:** Elderberry is known for its immune-boosting properties, which can indirectly support skin health by maintaining overall well-being.

10. Red Clover (Trifolium pratense):

- **Benefits:** Red clover is often used for its potential benefits in supporting hormonal balance, which can indirectly affect skin health.
- **Isoflavones:** Red clover contains isoflavones, compounds that may have estrogen-like effects.

11. Burdock Root (Arctium lappa):

- **Benefits:** Burdock root is believed to have detoxifying properties, helping to cleanse the blood and promote healthy skin.
- **Anti-Inflammatory:** Its anti-inflammatory properties may aid in managing skin conditions like acne and eczema.

12. Sarsaparilla (Smilax spp.):

- **Benefits:** Sarsaparilla is often associated with skin health due to its potential blood-purifying properties.
- **Detoxification:** Its detoxifying effects are thought to help address skin conditions by eliminating toxins from the body.

13. Irish Sea Moss (Chondrus crispus):

- **Benefits:** Irish sea moss, another type of seaweed, is rich in minerals and nutrients that may support overall health and skin radiance.
- **Mineral Content:** The minerals in sea moss can contribute to maintaining healthy skin cells.

14. Chaparral (Larrea tridentata):

- **Benefits:** Chaparral is traditionally used for its potential antimicrobial and anti-inflammatory effects on the skin.

- **Topical Use:** Chaparral can be used topically for its potential benefits in addressing skin issues.

15. Neem (Azadirachta indica):

- **Benefits:** Neem is often used in traditional Ayurvedic medicine for its potential antibacterial and anti-inflammatory properties.
- **Skin Health:** Neem oil and extracts can be used topically to support skin health and address various skin concerns.

16. Cascara Sagrada (Rhamnus purshiana):

- **Benefits:** Cascara sagrada is used for its potential laxative effects, which can contribute to detoxification and skin health.
- **Gentle Cleansing:** Proper elimination supports overall detoxification and can indirectly affect skin appearance.

17. Chickweed (Stellaria media):

- **Benefits:** Chickweed is often used for its soothing properties and potential benefits for dry, irritated skin.
- **Topical Use:** Chickweed can be used in skincare products or as a topical application for its potential calming effects.

18. Echinacea (Echinacea purpurea):

- **Benefits:** Echinacea is known for its immune-boosting properties, which can indirectly support skin health by maintaining overall well-being.

19. Chamomile (Matricaria chamomilla):

- **Benefits:** Chamomile is known for its calming and anti-inflammatory properties, which can benefit irritated or sensitive skin.
- **Topical Use:** Chamomile tea or chamomile-infused products can be used topically for skin comfort.

The Alkaline Diet for Glowing Skin

The alkaline diet is based on the concept that consuming foods that promote an alkaline pH in the body can improve overall health and well-being, including the appearance of the skin. This diet emphasizes the consumption of alkaline-forming foods while limiting acidic foods. The alkaline diet is thought to contribute to glowing skin by reducing inflammation, supporting detoxification, and providing essential nutrients. Here's a detailed explanation of how the alkaline diet can promote glowing skin:

1. Alkaline-Forming Foods:

- **Fruits and Vegetables:** These foods are rich in vitamins, minerals, and antioxidants that contribute to skin health and radiance.
- **Leafy Greens:** Kale, spinach, and other leafy greens provide nutrients like vitamin C, which supports collagen production.

2. Hydration:

- **Alkaline Water:** Drinking alkaline water may help maintain proper hydration levels and support overall skin health.

3. Reduced Inflammation:

- **Anti-Inflammatory Foods:** The diet focuses on whole foods that are naturally anti-inflammatory, potentially reducing skin inflammation.
- **Omega-3 Fatty Acids:** Alkaline foods like flaxseeds and walnuts provide omega-3 fatty acids, which can help reduce inflammation.

4. Acidic Foods Avoidance:

- **Limiting Acidic Foods:** Avoiding or reducing acidic foods like processed meats, sugary snacks, and excessive caffeine can help prevent skin inflammation.

5. Detoxification:

- **High-Fiber Foods:** Alkaline foods like fruits, vegetables, and whole grains are rich in fiber, which supports digestion and detoxification.

- **Detoxifying Enzymes:** Some alkaline foods contain enzymes that support the body's natural detox processes.

6. Antioxidant Intake:

- **Colorful Fruits and Vegetables:** These provide antioxidants like vitamins A, C, and E, which protect skin cells from oxidative stress.

7. Nutrient Support:

- **Vitamin and Mineral Rich:** Alkaline foods are often nutrient-dense, providing vitamins and minerals that support skin health.

8. Collagen Formation:

- **Vitamin C Intake:** Citrus fruits and other alkaline foods rich in vitamin C are important for collagen formation, which contributes to skin elasticity.

9. Balanced pH Levels:

- **Acidic Environment Impact:** High acidity in the body can contribute to inflammation, which may negatively affect skin health.
- **Alkaline Foods:** Consuming alkaline foods helps balance the body's pH levels, potentially benefiting skin health.

10. Avoiding Processed Foods:

- **Fresh Whole Foods:** The alkaline diet encourages the consumption of fresh, unprocessed foods that are nutrient-rich and support skin health.

11. Healthy Fats:

- **Avocado and Nuts:** Alkaline foods like avocados and nuts provide healthy fats that contribute to skin moisture and suppleness.

12. Maintaining Blood Sugar Levels:

- **Whole Grains:** Choosing alkaline whole grains like quinoa and brown rice helps maintain stable blood sugar levels, which can impact skin health.

13. Limiting Dairy and Sugar:

- **Dairy Alternatives:** The alkaline diet often suggests replacing dairy with plant-based alternatives, which may reduce the potential for skin issues related to dairy consumption.
- **Reduced Sugar Intake:** Minimizing sugar intake can help prevent glycation, a process that can contribute to skin aging.

14. Plant-Based Protein:

- **Legumes and Nuts:** Incorporate alkaline legumes like lentils and beans, as well as nuts and seeds, as sources of plant-based protein that support skin health.

15. Herbs and Spices:

- **Turmeric:** This anti-inflammatory spice, often included in the alkaline diet, may contribute to reducing skin inflammation and promoting radiance.

16. Alkaline Beverages:

- **Herbal Teas:** Herbal teas like chamomile, nettle, and green tea can provide antioxidants and hydration.

17. Mindful Eating:

- **Chewing Thoroughly:** Practicing mindful eating and chewing food thoroughly supports proper digestion and nutrient absorption, benefiting skin health.

18. Limiting Processed Foods:

- **Artificial Additives:** Minimizing processed foods reduces the intake of additives that can potentially impact skin health.

19. Individual Variability:

- **Personalized Approach:** Remember that everyone's skin and body respond differently to dietary changes, so it's important to find what works best for you.

20. Incorporate Variety:

- **Rainbow Diet:** Consume a variety of colorful fruits and vegetables to ensure a wide range of vitamins, minerals, and antioxidants.

21. Hydration:

- **Water Intake:** Alongside alkaline water, ensure you're drinking an adequate amount of plain water to support overall skin hydration.

22. Long-Term Lifestyle:

- **Sustainable Habits:** Focus on adopting long-term dietary habits that support both skin health and overall well-being.

23. Holistic Approach:

- **Comprehensive Care:** Combining the alkaline diet with other aspects of a healthy lifestyle, such as stress management and sleep, contributes to glowing skin.

24. Professional Guidance:

- **Registered Dietitian:** Seek guidance from a registered dietitian or healthcare professional to create a well-rounded dietary plan tailored to your individual needs.

25. Positive Mindset:

- **Confidence and Radiance:** Remember that feeling good about yourself and having a positive mindset can contribute to your skin's radiance.

26. Natural Skincare:

- **External Care:** Complement your alkaline diet with natural skincare products that suit your skin type and address specific concerns.

27. Sun Protection:

- **UV Exposure:** Protect your skin from the harmful effects of UV radiation by using sunscreen and minimizing sun exposure.

28. Consistency and Patience:

- **Timeframe:** Achieving glowing skin through dietary changes takes time, so be patient and stay consistent with your healthy habits.

29. Listening to Your Body:

- **Feedback:** Pay attention to how your skin responds to dietary changes and make adjustments as needed.

Embracing Skin Confidence: Nurturing Your True Beauty

True beauty comes from within, and embracing skin confidence involves more than just skincare routines and external practices. It's about cultivating self-love, self-acceptance, and a positive mindset that radiates from within. Here's a detailed explanation of how to nurture your true beauty and embrace skin confidence:

Self-Love and Acceptance:

Positive Self-Talk: Practice affirmations and replace self-criticism with self-compassion.

Celebrating Uniqueness: Embrace your individuality and appreciate the features that make you unique.

Mindful Self-Care:

Holistic Approach: Prioritize self-care practices that nourish your body, mind, and soul.

Regular Check-Ins: Take time to assess your needs and adjust your self-care routine accordingly.

Inner Wellness:

Nutrition: Focus on a balanced, nourishing diet that supports overall health and reflects on your skin's radiance.

Hydration: Drink enough water to stay hydrated and maintain skin's vitality.

Stress Management: Incorporate stress-reduction techniques like meditation, yoga, or deep breathing.

Quality Sleep: Prioritize sufficient and restful sleep for skin repair and rejuvenation.

Positive Body Image:

Appreciation: Focus on what your body does for you rather than how it looks.

Avoid Comparisons: Recognize that beauty standards are diverse and don't define your worth.

Limit Media Influence:

Selective Exposure: Choose media that promotes positive body image and self-esteem.

Reality Check: Remember that images often undergo editing and may not accurately reflect reality.

Empowerment:

Set Goals: Set achievable goals that align with your values and passions.

Celebrate Achievements: Acknowledge and celebrate your accomplishments, no matter how small.

Community Support:

Surround Yourself: Surround yourself with friends and loved ones who uplift and support you.

Connect: Engage with communities that foster body positivity and self-confidence.

Positive Rituals:

Mirror Work: Practice looking in the mirror and acknowledging your strengths and beauty.

Daily Affirmations: Incorporate daily affirmations that boost your confidence and self-esteem.

Wardrobe Choices:

Comfort and Expression: Wear clothes that make you feel comfortable and confident, expressing your unique style.

Authenticity: Dress for yourself rather than to meet others' expectations.

Professional Care:

Experts' Guidance: Seek professional help for skincare concerns or issues that impact your confidence.

Kindness and Gratitude:

Self-Care Habits: Approach self-care practices with kindness, seeing them as acts of self-love.

Gratitude: Cultivate gratitude for your body and the experiences it allows you to have.

Hobbies and Passions:

Nurturing Interests: Engage in activities you're passionate about, which can boost your self-esteem.

Authentic Relationships:

Boundaries: Set healthy boundaries to ensure your well-being and self-esteem in relationships.

Media Literacy:

Critical Thinking: Approach media messages with skepticism and evaluate their impact on your self-esteem.

Your Definition of Beauty:

Unique Perspective: Define beauty on your terms, based on your values and beliefs.

Growth Mindset:

Embrace Change: See challenges as opportunities for growth, resilience, and self-discovery.

Daily Affirmations:

Positive Declarations: Start your day with affirmations that boost your confidence and self-image.

Forgiveness:

Self-Compassion: Forgive yourself for any perceived flaws or mistakes, practicing self-compassion.

Appreciating Aging:

Natural Process: Embrace the natural aging process as a journey that adds to your beauty and wisdom.

Empathy and Kindness:

Spreading Positivity: Extend empathy and kindness to others, creating a positive environment.

Unplug and Reconnect:

Digital Detox: Take breaks from social media to reconnect with yourself and your surroundings.

Media Detox:

Mindful Consumption: Be conscious of media content you consume and its impact on your self-esteem.

Unfollow Negativity: Unfollow accounts or sources that promote unrealistic beauty standards or negativity.

Gratitude Journaling:

Daily Reflection: Keep a gratitude journal to focus on positive aspects of yourself and your life.

Volunteer and Give Back:

Helping Others: Volunteering and supporting others can boost your sense of purpose and confidence.

Body Positivity Movement:

Education: Learn about the body positivity movement to understand diverse definitions of beauty.

Focus on Strengths:

Strengths-Based Approach: Concentrate on your strengths, talents, and skills that make you unique.

Practice Self-Compassion:

Be Kind to Yourself: Treat yourself with the same kindness you extend to others.

Limit Negative Self-Talk:

Positive Language: Replace self-critical thoughts with positive affirmations and self-encouragement.

Visualization:

Positive Imagery: Practice visualizing yourself as confident, empowered, and radiating beauty.

Authentic Social Connections:

Meaningful Relationships: Nurture relationships that appreciate you for who you are, fostering self-confidence.

Celebrate Milestones:

Acknowledge Achievements: Celebrate your successes and milestones, reinforcing your self-worth.

Learn from Setbacks:

Resilience: View setbacks as opportunities to learn, grow, and become more resilient.

Practice Positivity:

Positivity Bias: Train your mind to focus on positive aspects and reframe challenges as opportunities.

Express Yourself:

Creativity: Engage in creative outlets that allow you to express yourself and boost self-esteem.

Personal Mantras:

Empowering Phrases: Create personal mantras that remind you of your worth and inner beauty.

Professional Growth:

Skill Development: Invest in learning and skill development, boosting your self-confidence.

Reflect and Adapt:

Personal Growth: Regularly reflect on your journey, adapt your approach, and celebrate progress.

Inspire Others:

Positive Influence: Your confidence and self-love can inspire others to embrace their true beauty.

Perception Shift:

Mind Over Matter: Focus on how you feel, think, and act rather than external perceptions.

Continuous Learning:

Self-Discovery: Embrace learning about yourself and your values throughout your life.

Book 13: Beating High Blood Pressure: Dr. Sebi's Guide to Hypertension Management

Understanding Hypertension: Causes and Risk Factors

Hypertension, commonly known as high blood pressure, is a chronic medical condition characterized by elevated blood pressure levels. Understanding the causes and risk factors associated with hypertension is crucial for its prevention, management, and overall well-being. Here's a detailed explanation of hypertension's causes and risk factors:

Understanding Blood Pressure:

- **Blood Pressure Measurement:** Blood pressure is measured in millimeters of mercury (mmHg) and consists of two values: systolic pressure (the top number) and diastolic pressure (the bottom number).
- **Normal Range:** Normal blood pressure is typically around 120/80 mmHg.

Causes of Hypertension:

1. Primary Hypertension:

- **Most Common:** Also known as essential hypertension, this form of high blood pressure develops gradually over time and doesn't have a specific underlying cause.
- **Lifestyle Factors:** Factors such as unhealthy diet, lack of exercise, stress, and genetics contribute to primary hypertension.

2. Secondary Hypertension:

- **Underlying Conditions:** Secondary hypertension is caused by an underlying medical condition, such as kidney disease, hormonal disorders, or certain medications.

Risk Factors for Hypertension:

1. Age:

- **Increased Risk:** The risk of developing hypertension increases with age. Blood vessels tend to become less flexible, contributing to higher blood pressure.

2. Family History:

- **Genetics:** A family history of hypertension increases the likelihood of developing the condition due to genetic factors.

3. Obesity:

- **Body Mass Index (BMI):** Excess body weight, especially when combined with an unhealthy diet, increases the risk of hypertension.
- **Visceral Fat:** Accumulation of fat around the abdomen (visceral fat) can contribute to insulin resistance and higher blood pressure.

4. Unhealthy Diet:

- **Sodium Intake:** Consuming high amounts of sodium, commonly found in processed and fast foods, can lead to fluid retention and increased blood pressure.
- **Low Potassium:** A diet low in potassium-rich foods can disrupt the balance of sodium and potassium, affecting blood pressure regulation.

5. Physical Inactivity:

- **Lack of Exercise:** Sedentary lifestyles contribute to weight gain and poor cardiovascular health, increasing the risk of hypertension.

6. Stress:

- **Chronic Stress:** Prolonged stress can lead to increased blood pressure due to hormonal and physiological responses.

7. Smoking:

- **Nicotine and Vasoconstriction:** Smoking narrows blood vessels and increases heart rate, raising blood pressure.

8. Alcohol Consumption:

- **Excessive Drinking:** Regular heavy alcohol consumption can lead to hypertension by damaging blood vessels and affecting the heart.

9. Chronic Kidney Disease:

- **Kidney Function:** Kidneys play a key role in regulating blood pressure. Dysfunction can lead to hypertension.

10. Diabetes:

- **Type 2 Diabetes:** People with diabetes are at an increased risk of hypertension due to insulin resistance and other metabolic factors.

11. Sleep Apnea:

- **Sleep Disordered Breathing:** Sleep apnea, characterized by interrupted breathing during sleep, is associated with hypertension.

12. Hormonal Factors:

- **Hormonal Imbalances:** Conditions like hyperthyroidism and certain hormonal disorders can contribute to hypertension.

13. Medications:

- **Certain Drugs:** Some medications, including birth control pills, decongestants, and nonsteroidal anti-inflammatory drugs (NSAIDs), can increase blood pressure.

14. Ethnicity:

- **Higher Prevalence:** Some ethnic groups, such as African Americans, have a higher prevalence of hypertension.

15. Gender:

- **Varied Patterns:** Hypertension patterns vary between men and women, with different risk factors playing a role.

16. Pregnancy-Related Hypertension:

- **Gestational Hypertension:** Some pregnant women develop high blood pressure during pregnancy, known as gestational hypertension.
- **Preeclampsia:** A more severe form of pregnancy-related hypertension, characterized by high blood pressure and organ damage.

17. Chronic Inflammation:

- **Inflammatory Markers:** Chronic inflammation, often linked to obesity and poor diet, can contribute to blood vessel damage and hypertension.

18. Socioeconomic Factors:

- **Access to Healthcare:** Limited access to medical care and resources can affect blood pressure management.
- Stress and Lifestyle: Socioeconomic factors can influence stress levels and lifestyle choices, contributing to hypertension.

19. Environmental Factors:

- **Air Pollution:** Exposure to air pollutants has been associated with higher blood pressure levels.

20. Salt Sensitivity:

- **Individual Variation:** Some individuals are more sensitive to the effects of dietary sodium, leading to higher blood pressure.

21. Hormone Imbalances:

- **Cushing's Syndrome:** An overproduction of cortisol, often due to adrenal gland disorders, can cause hypertension.
- **Primary Aldosteronism:** An excess of aldosterone hormone can lead to salt and water retention and elevated blood pressure.

22. Autoimmune Disorders:

- **Systemic Lupus Erythematosus (SLE):** Autoimmune conditions can affect blood vessel health and contribute to hypertension.

23. Caffeine Intake:

- **Stimulant Effect:** High caffeine intake, especially in sensitive individuals, can temporarily raise blood pressure.

24. Heavy Metal Exposure:

- **Lead and Cadmium:** Exposure to heavy metals like lead and cadmium has been linked to hypertension.

25. Poor Sleep Quality:

- **Sleep Duration and Quality:** Lack of adequate sleep and poor sleep quality can contribute to elevated blood pressure.

26. Overconsumption of Sugar:

- **Insulin Resistance:** Diets high in added sugars may contribute to insulin resistance and hypertension.

27. Chronic Alcohol Consumption:

- **Impact on Blood Pressure:** Long-term excessive alcohol consumption can lead to sustained high blood pressure.

28. Genetic Predisposition:

- **Family History:** Genetic factors can influence blood pressure regulation and predispose individuals to hypertension.

29. Lack of Nutrient Intake:

- **Vitamins and Minerals:** Deficiencies in nutrients like potassium, magnesium, and calcium can impact blood pressure regulation.

30. Blood Vessel Health:

- **Endothelial Dysfunction:** Damage to the inner lining of blood vessels can contribute to hypertension.

Dr. Sebi's Herbal Remedies for High Blood Pressure

Dr. Sebi, a renowned natural healer, advocated for holistic approaches to health and wellness. His herbal recommendations for high blood pressure focus on using natural ingredients to support the body's healing processes. It's important to note that while these herbal remedies are based on his teachings, individual responses may vary, and consulting a healthcare professional before making any changes to your treatment plan is advisable. Here's a detailed explanation of Dr. Sebi's herbal remedies for high blood pressure:

1. Celery Seed Extract:

- **Natural Diuretic:** Celery seed extract is believed to have diuretic properties, helping the body eliminate excess fluids and potentially reducing blood pressure.

2. Hawthorn Berry:

- **Cardiovascular Support:** Hawthorn berry is thought to support heart health and improve blood circulation, contributing to blood pressure regulation.

3. Garlic:

- **Vasodilation:** Garlic may promote blood vessel relaxation, leading to improved blood flow and potential blood pressure reduction.

4. Ginger:

- **Anti-Inflammatory:** Ginger's anti-inflammatory properties may contribute to blood vessel health and blood pressure management.

5. Cayenne Pepper:

- **Vasodilation:** Cayenne pepper is believed to promote vasodilation, which can lead to improved blood flow and potential blood pressure reduction.

6. Turmeric:

- **Anti-Inflammatory:** Turmeric's active compound, curcumin, has anti-inflammatory effects that could support overall cardiovascular health.

7. Dandelion:

- **Diuretic Properties:** Dandelion is thought to have diuretic effects, aiding in the elimination of excess fluids and potential blood pressure reduction.

8. Nettle Leaf:

- **Blood Vessel Health:** Nettle leaf may contribute to blood vessel health and overall cardiovascular function.

9. Olive Leaf:

- **Antioxidant Properties:** Olive leaf contains antioxidants that could protect blood vessels and support blood pressure regulation.

10. Soursop Leaf:

- **Natural Remedy:** Soursop leaves have been used in traditional medicine for various health benefits, including potential blood pressure support.

11. Burdock Root:

- **Detoxification:** Burdock root is believed to support detoxification processes, which could indirectly impact blood pressure.

12. Black Seed Oil:

- **Cardiovascular Health:** Black seed oil is thought to support heart health and blood pressure regulation.

13. Valerian Root:

- **Stress Reduction:** Valerian root's calming effects may indirectly contribute to blood pressure management by reducing stress.

14. Linden Flower:

- **Relaxation:** Linden flower is believed to have calming properties that could promote relaxation and potential blood pressure reduction.

15. Mistletoe:

- **Vasodilation:** Mistletoe is thought to promote blood vessel dilation, contributing to improved blood flow and potential blood pressure reduction.

16. Uva Ursi:

- **Diuretic Effects:** Uva ursi is believed to have diuretic properties that may aid in fluid elimination and potential blood pressure reduction.

17. Lemon Balm:

- **Calming Effects:** Lemon balm is believed to have calming properties that could indirectly contribute to blood pressure management by reducing stress.

18. Moringa:

- **Nutrient-Rich:** Moringa is rich in nutrients and antioxidants that may support overall cardiovascular health.

19. Bilberry:

- **Blood Vessel Support:** Bilberry's antioxidants and compounds may contribute to blood vessel health and blood pressure regulation.

20. Hibiscus Tea:

- **Blood Pressure Support:** Hibiscus tea has been studied for its potential to lower blood pressure due to its vasodilating effects.

21. Passionflower:

- **Stress Reduction:** Passionflower's calming effects may help lower stress levels, indirectly contributing to blood pressure management.

22. Ginkgo Biloba:

- **Circulation Improvement:** Ginkgo biloba is believed to support blood circulation, which can impact blood pressure regulation.

23. Oregano:

- **Antioxidant Properties:** Oregano contains antioxidants that may have positive effects on cardiovascular health.

24. Lavender:

- **Relaxation:** Lavender's soothing aroma may promote relaxation and stress reduction, indirectly benefiting blood pressure.

25. Motherwort:

- **Cardiovascular Support:** Motherwort has been used traditionally for heart health and could play a role in blood pressure regulation.

26. Ginseng:

- **Adaptogen:** Ginseng is an adaptogenic herb that may help the body adapt to stress, potentially impacting blood pressure.

27. Green Tea:

- **Antioxidant Content:** Green tea's antioxidants, particularly catechins, have been studied for their potential to support cardiovascular health.

28. Yarrow:

- **Blood Flow Improvement:** Yarrow may support blood vessel health and improve blood flow, contributing to blood pressure management.

29. Skullcap:

- **Nervous System Calming:** Skullcap's calming effects on the nervous system could indirectly impact blood pressure.

30. Chamomile:

- **Stress Reduction:** Chamomile's calming properties may help lower stress levels, which can have a positive effect on blood pressure.

31. Peppermint:

- **Vasodilation:** Peppermint may promote blood vessel relaxation, contributing to improved blood flow and potential blood pressure reduction.

32. Rosemary:

- **Antioxidant Content:** Rosemary's antioxidants may support overall cardiovascular health and blood pressure regulation.

33. Gymnema Sylvestre:

- **Blood Sugar Regulation:** Gymnema sylvestre may indirectly impact blood pressure by supporting blood sugar control.

34. Astragalus:

- **Adaptogenic Effects:** Astragalus is believed to have adaptogenic properties that could indirectly contribute to blood pressure management.

The Alkaline Diet for Blood Pressure Control

The alkaline diet, also known as the alkaline ash diet or alkaline acid diet, is based on the concept of consuming foods that help maintain a slightly alkaline pH level in the body. This diet emphasizes whole, natural foods that are believed to have an alkalizing effect on the body and promote overall health, including blood pressure regulation. Here's a detailed explanation of the alkaline diet's principles and its potential impact on blood pressure control:

Principles of the Alkaline Diet:

- **pH Balance:** The diet focuses on maintaining a slightly alkaline pH level in the body, which is believed to support various bodily functions.
- **Alkaline and Acidic Foods:** Foods are categorized as alkaline or acidic based on their

potential to influence the body's pH level.

- **High Alkaline Foods:** These include fruits, vegetables, nuts, seeds, and certain grains.
- **High Acidic Foods:** These include processed foods, animal products, refined sugars, and certain grains.

Impact on Blood Pressure:

1. Rich in Fruits and Vegetables:

- **Nutrient Density:** The alkaline diet emphasizes consuming a variety of fresh fruits and vegetables that are rich in vitamins, minerals, and antioxidants.
- **Potassium-Rich Foods:** Many alkaline foods, such as leafy greens, bananas, and avocados, are high in potassium, which is known to help regulate blood pressure.

2. Minimizes Processed Foods:

- **Sodium Reduction:** The diet discourages processed foods that are often high in sodium, which can contribute to high blood pressure.

3. Promotes Healthy Fats:

- **Healthy Fat Sources:** The diet encourages the consumption of healthy fats from sources like avocados, nuts, and seeds, which can support cardiovascular health.
- **Omega-3 Fatty Acids:** Alkaline foods like flaxseeds and walnuts provide omega-3 fatty acids that are associated with lower blood pressure.

4. Reduces Animal Products:

- **Lower Saturated Fat:** The diet reduces the intake of animal products, which can be high in saturated fat linked to cardiovascular issues, including high blood pressure.

5. Enhances Blood Vessel Health:

- **Antioxidant-Rich Foods:** Alkaline foods like berries and leafy greens contain antioxidants that support blood vessel health.

6. Incorporates Whole Grains:

- **Fiber Intake:** Whole grains like quinoa and brown rice provide fiber that may help regulate blood pressure.

7. Reduces Inflammatory Foods:

- **Anti-Inflammatory Benefits:** The diet's focus on natural, whole foods may help reduce inflammation, which can contribute to hypertension.

8. Hydration:

- **Importance of Water:** The alkaline diet emphasizes proper hydration, which is essential for blood pressure regulation.

9. Reduces Added Sugars:

- **Blood Sugar Management:** Minimizing added sugars can help manage blood sugar levels, which can affect blood pressure.

10. Stress Reduction:

- **Mindful Eating:** Practicing mindful eating as part of the alkaline diet can contribute to stress reduction, potentially impacting blood pressure.

11. Mindful Sodium Intake:

- **Monitor Salt Consumption:** While the alkaline diet encourages reducing processed foods that are high in sodium, it's important to be mindful of salt intake from other sources as well.

12. Adequate Hydration:

- **Water Intake:** Ensuring proper hydration is essential for maintaining healthy blood pressure levels and supporting overall cardiovascular health.

13. Portion Control:

- **Balanced Portions:** Pay attention to portion sizes to avoid overeating, as excess weight can contribute to high blood pressure.

14. Variety of Alkaline Foods:

- **Diverse Diet:** Aim for a variety of alkaline foods to ensure you receive a wide range of nutrients beneficial for blood pressure regulation.

15. Limiting Acidic Foods:

- **Moderation:** While acidic foods are not completely eliminated, practicing moderation with high acidic foods can help maintain pH balance.

16. Maintaining Nutrient Balance:

- **Balanced Nutrients:** Strive to maintain a balanced intake of carbohydrates, proteins, and healthy fats for optimal blood pressure control.

17. Consultation with a Healthcare Professional:

- **Individualized Guidance:** Seek advice from a healthcare professional or registered dietitian before making significant dietary changes, especially if you have pre-existing health conditions or are taking medications.

18. Consistency and Long-Term Approach:

- **Sustainable Habits:** Incorporate the principles of the alkaline diet into your lifestyle for the long term to experience lasting benefits for blood pressure control.

19. Regular Monitoring:

- **Blood Pressure Check:** Continue to monitor your blood pressure regularly and consult with a healthcare provider to track progress and make necessary adjustments.

20. Personalization:

- **Tailored Approach:** Every individual's nutritional needs and responses are unique. Customize the alkaline diet to suit your preferences, health status, and cultural considerations.

Lifestyle Strategies for Hypertension Management

Lifestyle plays a pivotal role in managing hypertension (high blood pressure). Implementing effective strategies can help lower blood pressure, reduce the risk of complications, and improve overall cardiovascular health. Here's a detailed explanation of lifestyle strategies for hypertension management:

1. Maintain a Balanced Diet:

- **DASH Diet:** The Dietary Approaches to Stop Hypertension (DASH) diet emphasizes fruits, vegetables, whole grains, lean proteins, and low-fat dairy products.
- **Sodium Reduction:** Limiting sodium intake by avoiding processed foods and using herbs and spices for flavoring can help manage blood pressure.
- **Potassium-Rich Foods:** Incorporate potassium-rich foods like bananas, oranges, potatoes, and spinach, as potassium helps balance sodium levels.
- **Magnesium-Rich Foods:** Foods like nuts, seeds, whole grains, and leafy greens are high in magnesium, which supports blood pressure regulation.

2. Regular Physical Activity:

- **Aerobic Exercise:** Engage in at least 150 minutes of moderate-intensity aerobic activity or 75 minutes of vigorous-intensity activity per week.
- **Strength Training:** Include muscle-strengthening exercises at least two days a week.
- **Beneficial Effects:** Regular exercise helps lower blood pressure, improve cardiovascular fitness, and maintain a healthy weight.

3. Weight Management:

- **Maintain a Healthy Weight:** Achieving and maintaining a healthy body weight can significantly contribute to blood pressure control.
- **Caloric Balance:** Create a balance between caloric intake and expenditure through a combination of diet and exercise.

4. Stress Management:

- **Relaxation Techniques:** Practice stress-reduction techniques such as deep breathing, meditation, yoga, or mindfulness to lower blood pressure.
- **Healthy Coping:** Adopt healthy ways to cope with stress, such as engaging in hobbies, spending time with loved ones, or engaging in physical activity.

5. Limit Alcohol Consumption:

- **Moderation:** If you drink alcohol, do so in moderation. For men, this generally means up to two drinks per day, and for women, up to one drink per day.
- **Excess Alcohol:** Excessive alcohol consumption can raise blood pressure and increase the risk of heart disease.

6. Quit Smoking:

- **Immediate Benefits:** Quitting smoking immediately improves blood pressure and reduces the risk of heart disease.
- **Support Resources:** Seek support from healthcare professionals, counseling, or support groups to successfully quit smoking.

7. Adequate Sleep:

- **Quality Sleep:** Aim for 7-9 hours of quality sleep each night to support blood pressure regulation and overall health.
- **Sleep Apnea:** If you suspect sleep apnea, seek medical evaluation and treatment.

8. Limit Caffeine Intake:

- **Moderation:** Consume caffeine in moderation, as excessive intake can temporarily elevate blood pressure.

9. Regular Blood Pressure Monitoring:

- **Home Monitoring:** Regularly monitor your blood pressure at home with a reliable blood pressure monitor.
- **Tracking Progress:** Keep a record of your readings and share them with your healthcare

provider.

10. Medication Adherence:

- **Follow Medical Advice:** If prescribed, take medication as directed by your healthcare provider.
- **Regular Check-Ups:** Attend regular medical appointments to monitor blood pressure and make necessary adjustments to medications.

11. Hydration:

- **Adequate Fluid Intake:** Drink plenty of water throughout the day to stay hydrated, as proper hydration supports blood pressure regulation.

12. Mindful Eating:

- **Slow and Mindful:** Practice mindful eating by chewing slowly, savoring each bite, and paying attention to hunger and fullness cues.

13. Limit Processed Foods:

- **Minimize Processed Foods:** Reduce the consumption of processed and fast foods that are often high in sodium, unhealthy fats, and added sugars.

14. Healthy Fats:

- **Choose Healthy Fats:** Opt for unsaturated fats from sources like avocados, nuts, seeds, and olive oil, as they support heart health.

15. Social Support:

- **Engage with Loved Ones:** Spending time with friends and family can provide emotional support and reduce stress, which positively impacts blood pressure.

16. Regular Health Check-Ups:

- **Routine Monitoring:** Regular medical check-ups help monitor blood pressure, assess overall health, and make informed decisions about treatment.

17. Limiting Screen Time:

- **Digital Detox:** Reduce screen time, especially before bedtime, to improve sleep quality and overall well-being.

18. Hygiene Practices:

- **Oral Health:** Proper dental care can help prevent gum disease, which is associated with higher blood pressure.

19. Limiting Artificial Sweeteners:

- **Moderation:** If using artificial sweeteners, do so in moderation, as some studies suggest they may impact blood pressure.

20. Cultural and Personal Considerations:

- **Cultural Foods:** Adapt your dietary choices to include traditional, culturally appropriate foods that align with hypertension management.

21. Mind-Body Practices:

- **Tai Chi and Yoga:** Mind-body practices like Tai Chi and yoga have been associated with stress reduction and blood pressure control.

22. Social Connection:

- **Community Engagement:** Participate in social or community activities to foster a sense of belonging and reduce isolation.

23. Environmental Factors:

- **Limit Exposure to Stressors:** Minimize exposure to environmental stressors and create a calming living environment.

24. Nutrition Label Awareness:

- **Read Labels:** Be mindful of nutrition labels to make informed choices about sodium, added sugars, and saturated fats.

25. Gradual Changes:

- **Sustainable Approach:** Implement changes gradually to make them more sustainable and easier to maintain over time.

26. Educational Resources:

- **Stay Informed:** Educate yourself about hypertension and its management through reputable sources and healthcare professionals.

27. Setting Realistic Goals:

- **Achievable Targets:** Set achievable goals for lifestyle changes, such as increasing physical activity or reducing sodium intake.

Book 14: Detoxify Your Body: Dr. Sebi's Cleansing and Detoxification Methods

The Importance of Detoxification for Health

Detoxification, often referred to as "detox," is a process that aims to eliminate harmful substances and toxins from the body. While the body has its own natural detoxification systems, there is a growing interest in various methods and practices to support and enhance these processes. Understanding the importance of detoxification for health involves recognizing how toxins can affect the body and exploring the ways in which detoxification practices may offer benefits. Here's a detailed explanation:

Toxins and Their Impact:

1. **Environmental Exposure:** We are exposed to toxins daily from the environment, including pollution, pesticides, heavy metals, and chemicals found in food, water, and the air.

2. **Processed Foods:** Processed and fast foods may contain additives, preservatives, and artificial flavors that contribute to toxin accumulation.

3. **Medications:** Certain medications and substances can introduce toxins or put stress on the body's detoxification systems.

4. **Stress and Lifestyle:** Chronic stress, lack of sleep, and poor lifestyle choices can hinder the body's ability to eliminate toxins effectively.

Importance of Detoxification:

1. **Enhanced Well-Being:** Detoxification aims to support the body's natural processes, allowing it to function optimally and maintain a sense of vitality.

2. **Reduced Toxin Load:** By facilitating the removal of toxins, detoxification may help reduce the overall toxic burden on the body.

3. **Improved Digestion:** Detox programs often involve consuming whole foods that are rich in fiber and nutrients, which can support digestive health.

4. **Boosted Energy Levels:** As the body eliminates toxins, individuals may experience increased energy and improved mental clarity.

5. **Weight Management:** Detox programs that focus on nutrient-dense foods can support healthy weight management by reducing consumption of processed foods and

promoting portion control.

6. **Support for Liver and Kidneys:** The liver and kidneys are key detoxification organs. Detox practices can potentially alleviate the strain on these organs.

7. **Skin Health:** Detoxification may lead to improved skin health by reducing the burden of toxins that can contribute to skin issues.

Types of Detoxification Practices:

1. **Nutrition-Based Detox:** These programs emphasize whole, nutrient-dense foods and encourage the elimination of processed foods, sugar, and unhealthy fats.

2. **Juice Cleanses:** Consuming fresh juices from fruits and vegetables for a designated period aims to provide nutrients while giving the digestive system a break.

3. **Fasting:** Intermittent fasting or extended fasting periods can allow the body to focus on cellular repair and detoxification.

4. **Herbal Support:** Certain herbs are believed to aid detoxification processes by supporting the liver, kidneys, and other organs.

5. **Hydration:** Drinking adequate water is crucial for proper detoxification, as it helps flush out toxins through urine and sweat.

6. **Sauna and Sweat Therapy:** Sweating through saunas, steam rooms, or exercise can help release toxins through the skin.

Considerations and Cautions:

1. **Individual Variability:** Each person's detoxification needs and responses are unique, and not all detox practices are suitable for everyone.

2. **Balanced Approach:** Extreme detoxification practices or prolonged fasting may lead to nutrient deficiencies and potential health risks.

3. **Consultation:** Before starting a detox program, it's important to consult a healthcare professional, especially if you have underlying health conditions or are taking medications.

4. **Sustainability:** Detox practices should be part of a balanced lifestyle, rather than a short-term fix.

Detoxification and Gut Health:

- **Gut-Body Connection:** Detox practices can positively impact gut health by promoting a diverse and balanced microbiome, which plays a crucial role in overall well-being.
- **Fiber-Rich Foods:** Consuming fiber-rich foods during detox can support gut health by nourishing beneficial gut bacteria.

Detox and Inflammation:

- **Reducing Inflammation:** Detoxification practices that emphasize anti-inflammatory foods may help reduce chronic inflammation, which is linked to various health issues.
- **Omega-3 Fatty Acids:** Foods rich in omega-3 fatty acids, such as fatty fish and flaxseeds, have anti-inflammatory properties that can support detoxification.

Detoxification and Mental Clarity:

- **Brain Health:** Some individuals report improved mental clarity and focus after detox programs, possibly due to reduced toxin load and improved nutrient intake.
- **Hydration and Brain Function:** Staying hydrated is vital for brain function, and detox practices often prioritize increased water intake.

Detoxification and Skin Health:

- **Clearer Skin:** Detoxification may lead to clearer and healthier skin by reducing the impact of toxins that can contribute to skin issues.
- **Hydration and Skin Radiance:** Proper hydration is key for maintaining skin elasticity and radiance.

Detox and Long-Term Health:

- **Preventing Chronic Diseases:** Detox practices that emphasize whole foods and nutrient-rich choices can potentially contribute to preventing chronic diseases.
- **Heart Health:** Detoxification can indirectly benefit cardiovascular health by promoting weight management, reducing inflammation, and supporting healthy blood pressure.

Detox as a Reset:

- **Starting Point:** Some individuals use detox programs as a reset to jump-start healthier habits and break from unhealthy patterns.
- **Education and Awareness:** Detox experiences can increase awareness about the impact of diet and lifestyle choices on health.

Adapting Detox Practices:

- **Personalization:** The ideal detox approach varies for each individual. Some people may benefit from short-term detoxes, while others may opt for ongoing dietary changes.

Professional Guidance:

- **Consult Healthcare Professionals:** Seek guidance from healthcare providers, registered dietitians, or certified nutritionists before embarking on any detox program, especially if you have underlying health conditions.

Mindful Approach:

- **Balance and Moderation:** Embrace detox practices in a balanced and moderate way, avoiding extreme or restrictive approaches.

Dr. Sebi's Herbal Detox Remedies

Dr. Sebi, also known as Alfredo Darrington Bowman, was a Honduran herbalist and natural healer who gained recognition for his holistic approach to health and wellness. He advocated for the use of natural plant-based foods and herbs to support the body's healing processes. Dr. Sebi's herbal detox remedies are based on his teachings and are intended to assist the body in its natural detoxification and healing processes. Here's a detailed explanation of some of his renowned herbal detox remedies:

1. Bladderwrack (Sea Moss):

- **Benefits:** Bladderwrack, also known as sea moss, is rich in minerals and nutrients that support thyroid function, immune health, and overall vitality.

2. Burdock Root:

- **Benefits:** Burdock root is known for its blood-purifying properties and its ability to support liver and kidney health. It may aid in detoxifying the blood and promoting healthy skin.

3. Dandelion:

- **Benefits:** Dandelion is often used to support liver and kidney function, aiding in the elimination of waste and toxins from the body.

4. Sarsaparilla:

- **Benefits:** Sarsaparilla is believed to cleanse the blood and support the body's natural detoxification processes. It's also used to promote healthy skin and joint health.

5. Yellow Dock:

- **Benefits:** Yellow dock is traditionally used to support liver function and promote healthy digestion. It may aid in detoxifying the body by assisting in the elimination of waste.

6. Elderberry:

- **Benefits:** Elderberry is known for its immune-boosting properties. It contains antioxidants that can aid in reducing oxidative stress and supporting overall wellness.

7. Bromide Plus Powder:

- **Benefits:** Dr. Sebi's Bromide Plus Powder is a blend of various herbs that are rich in bromine and other nutrients. It's intended to support thyroid health and aid in detoxification.

8. Chaparral:

- **Benefits:** Chaparral is used for its potential antimicrobial and antioxidant properties. It's believed to assist in detoxifying the body and supporting immune health.

9. Cascara Sagrada:

- **Benefits:** Cascara sagrada is a natural laxative that may support healthy bowel movements and aid in eliminating waste from the colon.

10. Irish Sea Moss:

- **Benefits:** Similar to bladderwrack, Irish sea moss is rich in minerals and nutrients that support thyroid health, immune function, and overall vitality.

11. Sage:

- **Benefits:** Sage is known for its antimicrobial properties and is often used to support respiratory health and detoxify the body.

12. Echinacea:

- **Benefits:** Echinacea is commonly used to support the immune system and may aid in reducing the severity and duration of colds and respiratory infections.

13. Red Clover:

- **Benefits:** Red clover is believed to support liver health and promote detoxification by assisting in the elimination of waste and toxins from the body.

14. African Bird Pepper:

- **Benefits:** African bird pepper is known for its potential digestive and circulatory benefits. It may aid in promoting circulation and digestion.

15. Bromide Plus Capsules:

- **Benefits:** Similar to the Bromide Plus Powder, the Bromide Plus Capsules contain a blend of herbs rich in bromine and other nutrients. They aim to support thyroid function and detoxification.

16. Wildcrafted Sea Moss Gel:

- **Benefits:** Sea moss gel is made from blending Irish moss (sea moss) with water. It's often used as a nutrient-rich addition to smoothies, desserts, or as a natural thickening agent.

17. Hemp Oil:

- **Benefits:** Hemp oil is rich in essential fatty acids and antioxidants that can support overall health, including skin health and immune function.

18. Bitter Melon:

- **Benefits:** Bitter melon is traditionally used to support blood sugar levels and promote healthy digestion. It may also aid in detoxifying the body.

19. Red Raspberry Leaf:

- **Benefits:** Red raspberry leaf is commonly used to support female reproductive health, but it also contains antioxidants that can contribute to overall wellness.

20. Valerian Root:

- **Benefits:** Valerian root is known for its potential calming and sedative effects, which can promote relaxation and stress reduction.

21. Guaco:

- **Benefits:** Guaco, also known as Mikania cordata, is used in traditional herbal medicine for its potential respiratory and immune-supporting properties.

22. Lily of the Valley:

- **Benefits:** Lily of the Valley is believed to support heart health and circulation. It's also used for its potential diuretic properties.

23. Gentian Root:

- **Benefits:** Gentian root is traditionally used to support digestive health and stimulate appetite. It may also aid in liver function.

24. Yellow Dock Root:

- **Benefits:** Yellow dock root is known for its potential liver-supporting properties. It may aid in detoxifying the body by promoting bile flow.

25. Lobelia:

- **Benefits:** Lobelia is believed to have potential respiratory and relaxation benefits. It's used in traditional herbal medicine for its various properties.

26. Cocolmeca:

- **Benefits:** Cocolmeca, also known as Smilax ornata, is traditionally used for its potential detoxification and blood-cleansing properties.

27. Bromide Mix:

- **Benefits:** Dr. Sebi's Bromide Mix is a blend of various herbs that are rich in bromine. It aims to support thyroid function and overall well-being.

The Alkaline Diet for Detoxification

The alkaline diet is a dietary approach that emphasizes consuming foods that have an alkaline-forming effect on the body, rather than an acidic one. Proponents of this diet believe that it can support detoxification by promoting a balanced pH level in the body and providing essential nutrients for optimal functioning. Here's a detailed explanation of the alkaline diet for detoxification:

1. Understanding Acid-Alkaline Balance:

- **pH Levels:** The body's pH level measures its acidity or alkalinity on a scale of 0 to 14. A pH level of 7 is considered neutral, while levels below 7 are acidic and levels above 7 are alkaline.
- **Alkaline Forming Foods:** Alkaline-forming foods include fruits, vegetables, nuts, seeds, and certain grains. These foods are believed to help maintain a slightly alkaline pH in the body.
- **Acid-Forming Foods:** Acid-forming foods, such as processed foods, animal proteins, and refined sugars, are believed to contribute to acidity in the body.

2. Benefits of the Alkaline Diet for Detoxification:

- **Balanced pH Levels:** Proponents of the alkaline diet suggest that consuming more alkaline-forming foods can help balance the body's pH levels and promote overall well-being.
- **Nutrient Intake:** The diet encourages the consumption of nutrient-rich foods, such as fruits and vegetables, which provide vitamins, minerals, and antioxidants that support detoxification.
- **Hydration:** Many alkaline-forming foods are also hydrating, such as water-rich fruits and vegetables, which can support the body's natural detoxification processes.
- **Reduced Processed Foods:** The alkaline diet discourages processed foods that may contribute to acidity in the body and promote the consumption of whole, unprocessed foods.

3. Alkaline and Acidic Foods:

- **Alkaline-Forming Foods:** Include a variety of fresh fruits, vegetables (e.g., leafy greens, broccoli, cucumbers), nuts, seeds (e.g., almonds, chia seeds), and legumes (e.g., lentils, beans).
- **Moderate Acid-Forming Foods:** Some foods, such as whole grains (e.g., quinoa, brown rice), can be included in moderation without significantly affecting the body's pH levels.
- **Limit Acid-Forming Foods:** Limit or avoid foods that are highly acid-forming, including processed foods, sugary beverages, animal meats, dairy products, and refined sugars.

4. Meal Planning for Detoxification:

- **Plant-Based Emphasis:** Plan meals around plant-based foods like colorful vegetables, leafy greens, fruits, and whole grains.
- **Variety:** Incorporate a variety of alkaline-forming foods to ensure a balanced nutrient intake.
- **Hydration:** Stay hydrated with water, herbal teas, and water-rich fruits like watermelon and oranges.
- **Lean Proteins:** If desired, choose plant-based protein sources like legumes, lentils, quinoa, and tofu.

5. Limitations and Considerations:

- **Scientific Evidence:** While the alkaline diet's principles align with consuming nutrient-rich foods, there is limited scientific evidence supporting its direct impact on detoxification or pH balance.
- **Individual Variability:** The body's ability to regulate pH levels is complex, and individual responses to the diet may vary.
- **Balanced Approach:** It's important to avoid extreme restrictions and ensure a balanced intake of all essential nutrients.
- **Consultation:** Before making significant dietary changes, consult with a healthcare professional or registered dietitian, especially if you have underlying health conditions.

6. Antioxidant-Rich Foods:

- **Berries:** Blueberries, strawberries, and other berries are rich in antioxidants that can help neutralize harmful free radicals and support detoxification.
- **Leafy Greens:** Greens like kale, spinach, and Swiss chard are not only alkaline-forming but also packed with vitamins, minerals, and antioxidants.
- **Citrus Fruits:** Lemons, limes, and grapefruits are acidic in nature but have an alkalizing effect on the body due to their mineral content. They also support liver function.

7. Hydration and Detoxification:

- **Water:** Staying adequately hydrated is crucial for detoxification. Water helps flush out toxins through urine, supports digestion, and maintains overall bodily functions.
- **Herbal Teas:** Herbal teas like dandelion root, nettle, and ginger can support detoxification by promoting healthy liver and kidney function.

8. Fiber-Rich Foods:

- **Whole Grains:** While some whole grains are considered slightly acid-forming, they still provide essential fiber that supports digestion and helps eliminate waste.
- **Legumes:** Beans, lentils, and chickpeas are excellent sources of fiber that aid in promoting regular bowel movements and supporting gut health.

9. Mindful Eating Practices:

- **Chewing Slowly:** Chewing food thoroughly supports proper digestion and absorption of nutrients, enhancing the body's ability to eliminate waste effectively.
- **Portion Control:** Practicing portion control helps prevent overeating and supports digestion, allowing the body to focus on detoxification.

10. Avoiding Processed Foods:

- **Processed Foods:** Highly processed foods, such as sugary snacks, fast food, and processed meats, can contribute to acidity and inflammation in the body.
- **Added Sugars:** Minimize the consumption of foods and beverages high in added sugars, as excessive sugar intake can hinder detoxification processes.

11. Sustainable Approach:

- **Long-Term Habits:** Instead of viewing the alkaline diet as a short-term detox, consider adopting its principles as a long-term dietary approach for overall health.

12. Personalization:

- **Individual Needs:** Tailor the alkaline diet to your individual preferences, nutritional needs, and health goals. What works for one person may not work the same way for another.

13. Monitoring Changes:

- **Self-Observation:** Pay attention to how your body responds to dietary changes. Monitor energy levels, digestion, skin health, and overall well-being.

14. Comprehensive Wellness:

- **Holistic Approach:** While the alkaline diet can be a component of a healthy lifestyle, remember that overall wellness also includes stress management, regular physical activity, and adequate sleep.

Conclusion:

The alkaline diet for detoxification centers on consuming alkaline-forming foods to promote a balanced pH and support the body's natural detoxification processes. While the diet emphasizes nutrient-rich plant foods, it's important to approach it as part of a broader holistic approach to health. By focusing on hydration, consuming antioxidant-rich foods, practicing mindful eating, and avoiding processed foods, you can create a nourishing and supportive environment for your body's detoxification processes. Remember that individual responses to dietary changes vary, and it's advisable to consult with healthcare professionals or registered dietitians before making significant dietary shifts, especially if you have underlying health conditions. Incorporating the principles of the alkaline diet alongside other healthy lifestyle habits can contribute to your overall well-being.

Book 15: Boosting Immune Power: Dr. Sebi's Natural Solutions for a Strong Immune System

Understanding the Immune System and its Functions

The immune system is a complex network of cells, tissues, and organs that work together to defend the body against harmful pathogens, such as viruses, bacteria, fungi, and other foreign invaders. It plays a vital role in maintaining health and protecting the body from infections and diseases. Here's a detailed explanation of the immune system's functions, components, and mechanisms:

1. Components of the Immune System:

- **White Blood Cells (Leukocytes):** White blood cells are the primary defenders of the immune system. They include various types, such as neutrophils, lymphocytes (T cells and B cells), monocytes, eosinophils, and basophils.
- **T Cells:** T cells play a key role in cellular immunity. They recognize and destroy infected or abnormal cells directly.
- **B Cells:** B cells are responsible for producing antibodies, proteins that target specific pathogens. Antibodies bind to pathogens, marking them for destruction by other immune cells.
- **Antibodies (Immunoglobulins):** Antibodies are Y-shaped proteins produced by B cells. They neutralize pathogens by binding to them, preventing them from infecting cells.
- **Macrophages:** Macrophages are large white blood cells that engulf and digest pathogens, dead cells, and debris.
- **Natural Killer (NK) Cells:** NK cells are responsible for identifying and destroying infected cells and cancerous cells.
- **Complement System:** A group of proteins that help antibodies and phagocytes eliminate pathogens more effectively.
- **Lymphatic System:** A network of vessels, nodes, and organs that transports lymph (a clear fluid containing white blood cells) and helps filter and trap pathogens.

2. Functions of the Immune System:

- **Recognition:** The immune system identifies self-cells and non-self cells (pathogens) by recognizing specific molecules on their surfaces.

233

- **Neutralization:** Antibodies bind to pathogens, preventing them from entering or infecting host cells.
- **Phagocytosis:** Phagocytes, including macrophages and neutrophils, engulf and digest pathogens, debris, and dead cells.
- **Cellular Immunity:** T cells recognize and directly attack infected or abnormal cells.
- **Humoral Immunity:** B cells produce antibodies that neutralize pathogens in body fluids.
- **Memory Response:** After an initial encounter with a pathogen, the immune system retains memory cells (memory T cells and memory B cells) that allow for a rapid and effective response upon re-exposure to the same pathogen.
- **Inflammation:** Inflammatory response involves increased blood flow, dilation of blood vessels, and recruitment of immune cells to the site of infection or injury.

3. Types of Immune Responses:

- **Innate Immunity:** This is the first line of defense and includes physical barriers (skin), chemicals (stomach acid), and innate immune cells (neutrophils, macrophages) that provide rapid but non-specific responses.
- **Adaptive Immunity:** This is the second line of defense and involves the recognition of specific pathogens. It includes B cells and T cells that produce tailored responses against specific antigens.

4. Immune Disorders:

- **Autoimmune Diseases:** In autoimmune diseases, the immune system mistakenly attacks the body's own cells and tissues, causing conditions like rheumatoid arthritis, lupus, and multiple sclerosis.
- **Immunodeficiency Disorders:** Immunodeficiency disorders result in a weakened or absent immune response, making individuals more susceptible to infections. Examples include HIV/AIDS and primary immunodeficiency disorders.
- **Allergies:** Allergies occur when the immune system reacts excessively to harmless substances, leading to symptoms like sneezing, itching, and hives.

5. Factors Influencing Immune Function:

- **Nutrition:** Adequate intake of vitamins, minerals, antioxidants, and protein supports immune function.

- **Sleep:** Quality sleep is essential for immune system maintenance and responsiveness.
- **Stress:** Chronic stress can suppress the immune system, making the body more vulnerable to infections.
- **Physical Activity:** Regular exercise promotes overall health, circulation, and immune function.
- **Age:** Immune function changes over the lifespan, with the elderly and very young being more susceptible to infections.
- **Vaccination:** Vaccines stimulate the immune system to create a memory response without causing the disease itself.

6. Antigen Presentation:

- **Antigen-Presenting Cells (APCs):** Dendritic cells, macrophages, and B cells capture antigens from pathogens and present them to T cells for recognition.
- **Major Histocompatibility Complex (MHC):** MHC molecules on APCs present antigens to T cells, allowing them to distinguish between self and non-self cells.

7. Cytokines:

- **Cell Signaling Proteins:** Cytokines are proteins that facilitate communication between immune cells, regulating their activities and responses.
- **Interleukins:** Interleukins play a role in inflammation, immune cell activation, and communication between different immune cells.
- **Chemokines:** Chemokines guide immune cells to sites of infection or inflammation.

8. Immune Memory:

- **Memory Cells:** Memory T cells and memory B cells are long-lived cells that "remember" specific pathogens. This allows for a faster and more effective response upon re-exposure.

9. Cross-Reactivity:

- **Cross-Reactive Immunity:** Sometimes, the immune response generated against one pathogen can provide some degree of protection against related pathogens.

10. Tolerance:

- **Immune Tolerance:** The immune system is designed to recognize and tolerate the body's own cells and tissues to prevent autoimmune reactions.

11. Immunization and Vaccination:

- **Vaccines:** Vaccination involves introducing a harmless form of a pathogen or its antigens into the body to stimulate the immune system's memory response. This provides protection against future infections.

12. Immunosenescence:

- **Aging and Immunity:** Immunosenescence refers to the gradual decline in immune function that occurs with age, making older individuals more susceptible to infections and less responsive to vaccines.

13. Immunotherapy:

- **Cancer Immunotherapy:** Immunotherapy uses the body's immune system to target and destroy cancer cells. This includes immune checkpoint inhibitors and CAR-T cell therapy.

14. Immunodeficiency Disorders:

- **Primary Immunodeficiencies:** These are genetic disorders that result in a weakened immune system from birth.
- **Acquired Immunodeficiencies:** Conditions like HIV/AIDS lead to a compromised immune system due to infection by the human immunodeficiency virus.

15. Allergic Reactions:

- **Allergens:** Allergic reactions occur when the immune system overreacts to harmless substances, releasing histamines and causing symptoms like itching, sneezing, and hives.

16. Autoimmune Diseases:

- **Loss of Self-Tolerance:** Autoimmune diseases occur when the immune system mistakenly targets and attacks the body's own cells and tissues.

17. Inflammation and Immunity:

- **Inflammatory Response:** Inflammation is a protective response to infections or injuries, involving increased blood flow and immune cell activity.
- **Chronic Inflammation:** Prolonged or excessive inflammation can lead to chronic diseases like cardiovascular disease and diabetes.

18. Future of Immune Research:

- **Personalized Medicine:** Advancements in immune research are leading to personalized treatments based on an individual's immune profile.
- **Emerging Therapies:** New approaches, such as using CRISPR technology to modify immune cells, are being explored for treating various diseases.

19. Maintaining Immune Health:

- **Balanced Diet:** A diet rich in fruits, vegetables, lean proteins, and healthy fats supports immune function.
- **Hygiene:** Proper hygiene practices, including handwashing, help prevent infections.
- **Stress Management:** Managing stress through relaxation techniques, exercise, and social support benefits immune health.
- **Avoiding Overuse of Antibiotics:** Overuse of antibiotics can lead to antibiotic resistance and compromise immune response.

Dr. Sebi's Immune-Enhancing Herbs and Practices

Dr. Sebi, a renowned herbalist and natural healer, advocated for a holistic approach to health and believed in using natural, plant-based remedies to enhance the immune system. His teachings emphasized the importance of maintaining an alkaline body pH and supporting the body's ability to heal itself. Here's a detailed explanation of some of the immune-enhancing herbs and practices recommended by Dr. Sebi:

1. Irish Sea Moss (Chondrus Crispus):

- **Rich in Nutrients:** Irish sea moss is abundant in vitamins, minerals, and trace elements that support immune function and overall health.
- **Antiviral Properties:** It is believed to have antiviral properties that can help protect against infections.
- **Alkalizing:** Irish sea moss is alkaline in nature, which can contribute to balancing the body's pH levels.

2. Elderberry (Sambucus Nigra):

- **Antioxidant-Rich:** Elderberry is rich in antioxidants, which help combat oxidative stress and support immune health.
- **Antiviral Activity:** Elderberry is known for its potential antiviral effects, particularly against certain strains of the flu virus.

3. Burdock Root (Arctium Lappa):

- **Detoxification:** Burdock root is believed to support detoxification, which can help remove toxins and promote a healthier immune system.
- **Anti-Inflammatory:** It has anti-inflammatory properties that may aid in reducing inflammation in the body.

4. Bladderwrack (Fucus Vesiculosus):

- **Rich in Iodine:** Bladderwrack contains iodine, which is essential for thyroid function and overall immune support.

- **Mineral-Rich:** It is a source of various minerals that contribute to overall health and immune function.

5. Sarsaparilla Root (Smilax Officinalis):

- **Blood Purification:** Sarsaparilla root is believed to purify the blood and support overall detoxification.
- **Anti-Inflammatory:** Its anti-inflammatory properties may help reduce inflammation and promote immune balance.

6. Dandelion (Taraxacum Officinale):

- **Liver Support:** Dandelion is thought to support liver health, aiding in detoxification and immune function.
- **Rich in Vitamins:** It is a source of vitamins A, C, and E, which are important for immune support.

7. Echinacea (Echinacea Purpurea):

- **Immune Modulation:** Echinacea is believed to modulate the immune system, enhancing its response to infections.
- **Antiviral and Antibacterial:** It is thought to have antiviral and antibacterial properties that can help fight off pathogens.

8. Burdock Root (Arctium Lappa):

- **Detoxification:** Burdock root is believed to support detoxification, which can help remove toxins and promote a healthier immune system.
- **Anti-Inflammatory:** It has anti-inflammatory properties that may aid in reducing inflammation in the body.

9. Chaparral (Larrea Tridentata):

- **Antioxidant:** Chaparral is rich in antioxidants that can protect cells from oxidative damage and support immune function.
- **Antiviral and Antibacterial:** It is believed to have antiviral and antibacterial properties that can help fight infections.

10. Alkaline Diet:

- **Plant-Based:** Dr. Sebi emphasized a plant-based diet consisting of alkaline foods, such as fruits, vegetables, nuts, seeds, and grains.
- **Avoiding Acidic Foods:** He recommended avoiding acidic foods like processed foods, dairy, refined sugars, and animal products.

11. Hydration:

- **Water Intake:** Staying well-hydrated is essential for maintaining bodily functions and supporting immune health.

12. Rest and Stress Management:

- **Adequate Sleep:** Getting sufficient rest allows the body to regenerate and supports immune function.
- **Stress Reduction:** Managing stress through relaxation techniques, meditation, and deep breathing can help maintain a strong immune system.

13. Physical Activity:

- **Regular Exercise:** Engaging in regular physical activity supports overall health and immune function.

14. Sunlight Exposure:

- **Vitamin D Synthesis:** Sunlight exposure helps the body produce vitamin D, which plays a crucial role in immune health.

15. Positive Mindset:

- **Mental Well-Being:** Cultivating a positive mindset and reducing negative stressors can support overall immune function.

16. Herbal Teas:

- **Immune-Boosting Herbal Blends:** Dr. Sebi's recommendations may include various herbal teas, such as ginger, echinacea, elderberry, and pau d'arco, which are known for their potential immune-enhancing properties.

- **Antioxidant Support:** Many of these herbs are rich in antioxidants, which can help protect cells from oxidative stress and support immune health.

17. Fasting:

- **Intermittent Fasting:** Dr. Sebi's approach might involve intermittent fasting, which allows the body to focus on repair and immune function during periods of fasting.
- **Detoxification:** Fasting can promote detoxification, allowing the body to eliminate waste and toxins.

18. Colon Cleansing:

- **Eliminating Toxins:** Dr. Sebi emphasized the importance of colon cleansing to remove accumulated waste and toxins, supporting overall health and immune function.

19. Alkaline Electrolyte Drinks:

- **Hydration and Electrolytes:** Alkaline electrolyte drinks, made with ingredients like Irish sea moss and fruits, can help maintain hydration and provide essential electrolytes.
- **Electrolyte Balance:** Proper electrolyte balance is important for cellular functions and immune response.

20. Avoiding Harmful Substances:

- **Processed Foods:** Dr. Sebi recommended avoiding processed and refined foods, which can contribute to inflammation and weaken the immune system.
- **Artificial Additives:** He emphasized avoiding artificial additives, preservatives, and chemicals that may negatively impact immune health.

21. Plant-Based Supplements:

- **Natural Supplements:** Dr. Sebi's approach may include plant-based supplements, such as bladderwrack capsules, elderberry extracts, and other natural products.
- **Supporting Immune Health:** These supplements can provide additional support to the immune system when used as part of a holistic approach.

22. Avoiding Overexertion:

- **Balanced Activity:** Dr. Sebi's philosophy suggests avoiding excessive physical and mental strain, allowing the body to conserve energy for immune function.

23. Mindful Eating:

- **Chewing Thoroughly:** Dr. Sebi encouraged chewing food thoroughly to aid digestion and nutrient absorption.
- **Mindful Consumption:** Paying attention to what and how you eat supports proper digestion and nutrient utilization.

24. Detoxifying Baths:

- **Epsom Salt Baths:** Detoxifying baths, using ingredients like Epsom salts, can promote relaxation, enhance circulation, and aid in detoxification.

25. Herbal Poultices and Compresses:

- **Localized Application:** Dr. Sebi's approach might involve using herbal poultices or compresses on specific areas to support healing and immune function.

26. Affirmations and Positive Thoughts:

- **Mind-Body Connection:** Dr. Sebi recognized the importance of positive thoughts and affirmations in promoting a healthy mind-body connection.
- **Stress Reduction:** Practicing positive self-talk and affirmations can contribute to stress reduction and immune support.

27. Caring for the Lymphatic System:

- **Lymphatic Massage:** Dr. Sebi's recommendations may include practices like lymphatic massage to support lymphatic circulation and immune health.
- **Fluid Balance:** A healthy lymphatic system contributes to fluid balance and immune cell transport.

28. Nature and Fresh Air:

- **Connection with Nature:** Spending time outdoors and enjoying fresh air can promote relaxation and reduce stress, benefiting immune health.

29. Holistic Well-Being:

- **Mind, Body, and Spirit:** Dr. Sebi's approach to immune enhancement emphasizes the interconnectedness of the mind, body, and spirit.
- **Holistic Health:** By nurturing all aspects of well-being, including emotional, mental, and spiritual aspects, individuals can support immune function and overall vitality.

The Alkaline Diet for Optimal Immune Function

The alkaline diet is based on the concept of consuming foods that promote an alkaline pH in the body, which is believed to support overall health, including immune function. This diet emphasizes a higher intake of alkaline-forming foods and a reduction in acid-forming foods. Here's a detailed explanation of the alkaline diet's principles and its potential impact on immune function:

1. Alkaline-Forming Foods:

- **Fresh Fruits:** Most fruits, such as berries, citrus fruits, melons, and apples, are alkaline-forming and rich in vitamins, minerals, antioxidants, and fiber that support immune health.
- **Vegetables:** Leafy greens, cruciferous vegetables (broccoli, cauliflower), root vegetables (sweet potatoes, carrots), and others are alkaline and provide essential nutrients for immune function.
- **Nuts and Seeds:** Almonds, chia seeds, and flaxseeds are alkaline and contain healthy fats, proteins, and antioxidants that benefit immune health.
- **Herbs and Spices:** Many herbs and spices, including ginger, turmeric, and garlic, are alkaline and known for their immune-enhancing properties.

2. Acidic Foods to Limit:

- **Processed Foods:** Processed foods often contain additives, sugars, and unhealthy fats that can promote inflammation and weaken the immune system.
- **Animal Products:** Meat, dairy, and other animal products are generally acid-forming and may contribute to an acidic body environment.
- **Refined Sugars:** Refined sugars can lead to inflammation and compromise immune function.

3. Hydration:

- **Alkaline Water:** Consuming alkaline water is recommended on the alkaline diet to help maintain proper body pH and support hydration.

4. Benefits for Immune Function:

- **Anti-Inflammatory:** Alkaline-forming foods tend to be anti-inflammatory, which can help modulate the immune response and reduce chronic inflammation.
- **Nutrient-Rich:** Alkaline foods are often nutrient-dense, providing vitamins (A, C, E), minerals (magnesium, potassium), and antioxidants that enhance immune function.
- **Gut Health:** The diet's emphasis on plant-based foods can promote a healthy gut microbiome, which plays a role in immune regulation.

5. Avoiding Excess Acid Load:

- **Acid Load:** Excessive consumption of acidic foods may increase the body's acid load, potentially impacting immune response and overall health.

6. Alkaline Diet and Chronic Diseases:

- **Preventing Chronic Diseases:** The alkaline diet's focus on whole, plant-based foods is associated with a reduced risk of chronic diseases, which can indirectly support immune function.

7. Balanced Approach:

- **Variety:** Consuming a variety of alkaline-forming foods ensures a well-rounded intake of nutrients that support the immune system.

8. Potential Limitations:

- **Individual Responses:** The alkaline diet's impact on immune function can vary among individuals based on genetics, lifestyle, and underlying health conditions.

9. Consultation with Professionals:

- **Healthcare Provider:** It's important to consult a healthcare provider or registered dietitian before making significant dietary changes, especially if you have existing health conditions.

10. Meal Planning for Immune Support:

- **Colorful Plates:** Aim to have a variety of colorful fruits and vegetables on your plate. Different colors indicate a range of antioxidants and nutrients that support immune health.
- **Whole Grains:** Incorporate whole grains like quinoa, brown rice, and oats for sustained energy and fiber that supports gut health.
- **Plant-Based Proteins:** Opt for plant-based protein sources like beans, lentils, chickpeas, and tofu. These foods provide essential amino acids without the acidity of animal products.
- **Healthy Fats:** Include sources of healthy fats such as avocados, nuts, seeds, and olive oil. Omega-3 fatty acids found in flaxseeds and chia seeds are particularly beneficial for immune function.

11. Balancing Acidic and Alkaline Foods:

- **Moderation:** While the alkaline diet encourages reducing acidic foods, you don't need to completely eliminate them. It's about balance and overall patterns of consumption.

12. Meal Timing:

- **Regular Meals:** Aim for regular, balanced meals throughout the day to provide a consistent supply of nutrients to support immune health.
- **Intermittent Fasting:** If considering intermittent fasting, consult with a healthcare

professional to ensure it's appropriate for your health and immune needs.

13. Incorporating Alkaline Beverages:

- **Herbal Teas:** Herbal teas like ginger, turmeric, and echinacea can complement an alkaline diet and provide additional immune-boosting properties.
- **Alkaline Water:** Drinking alkaline water can help maintain a proper body pH and support hydration.

14. Avoiding Processed Foods:

- **Read Labels:** Avoid highly processed foods that often contain artificial additives, high levels of sodium, and unhealthy fats that can negatively impact immune health.

15. Food Preparation:

- **Raw vs. Cooked:** Incorporate a mix of raw and cooked vegetables. Some nutrients are better absorbed when foods are cooked, while others are more bioavailable when consumed raw.
- **Food Safety:** Proper food handling and hygiene are essential to prevent foodborne illnesses that can compromise immune function.

16. Mindful Eating:

- **Slow Down:** Practice mindful eating by chewing food thoroughly and savoring each bite. This aids digestion and nutrient absorption.
- **Stress Reduction:** Reducing stress during mealtime supports optimal digestion and nutrient utilization.

17. Individualization:

- **Personalized Approach:** What works for one person may not work for another. Listen to your body and adjust your diet based on your individual responses.

18. Long-Term Lifestyle Choice:

- **Sustainable Approach:** The alkaline diet is most effective when adopted as a long-term lifestyle choice rather than a short-term fix.

19. Comprehensive Immune Support:

- **Holistic Approach:** While the alkaline diet can contribute to immune health, it's important to combine it with other immune-boosting practices like stress management, sleep, exercise, and hygiene.

20. Professional Guidance:

- **Healthcare Provider:** Consult with a healthcare provider or registered dietitian before making significant dietary changes, especially if you have existing health conditions or concerns.

Conclusion:

The alkaline diet's focus on nutrient-dense, plant-based foods aligns with supporting optimal immune function. By prioritizing alkaline-forming foods and minimizing acidic choices, you can provide your body with essential nutrients, antioxidants, and a balanced pH environment that contributes to a robust immune system. However, remember that the alkaline diet should be part of a holistic approach to health that includes other immune-enhancing practices and a healthy lifestyle. It's important to tailor dietary choices to your individual needs, seek professional guidance, and make informed decisions that support your immune health in the long term.

Lifestyle Strategies to Support Immunity

In addition to dietary choices, certain lifestyle strategies play a crucial role in supporting immune function and overall health. These strategies encompass a range of practices that contribute to a strong immune system and overall well-being. Here's a detailed explanation of various lifestyle strategies to consider:

Adequate Sleep:

Quality Rest: Aim for 7-9 hours of quality sleep each night. Sleep is essential for immune system repair, cell regeneration, and overall health.

Consistent Schedule: Establish a consistent sleep schedule by going to bed and waking up at the same times each day.

Stress Management:

Relaxation Techniques: Practice relaxation methods such as deep breathing, meditation, yoga, and mindfulness to reduce stress.

Hobbies: Engage in activities you enjoy to relieve stress and promote a positive mood.

Regular Physical Activity:

Moderate Exercise: Engage in regular moderate exercise, such as walking, jogging, cycling, or swimming, to support circulation and immune function.

Strength Training: Incorporate strength training to build muscle and enhance overall fitness.

Hygiene and Sanitation:

Handwashing: Regularly wash hands with soap and water for at least 20 seconds to prevent the spread of pathogens.

Proper Food Handling: Adhere to safe food handling practices to prevent foodborne illnesses.

Stay Hydrated:

Adequate Fluid Intake: Drink plenty of water and hydrating beverages throughout the day to support bodily functions and immune response.

Limit Alcohol and Tobacco:

Moderation: If consuming alcohol, do so in moderation. Excessive alcohol intake can weaken the immune system.

Avoid Smoking: Avoid smoking and exposure to secondhand smoke, as they can impair immune function.

Sunlight Exposure:

Vitamin D Synthesis: Spend time in the sun to allow your body to produce vitamin D, which plays a role in immune health.

Protect Skin: Be mindful of sun protection to avoid excessive UV exposure.

Mindfulness and Relaxation:

Mind-Body Connection: Engage in mindfulness practices like meditation, deep breathing, and progressive muscle relaxation to manage stress and promote immune health.

Social Connections:

Meaningful Relationships: Maintain strong social connections with friends and family to support mental and emotional well-being.

Support System: A robust support system contributes to lower stress levels and better immune function.

Positive Outlook:

Positive Mindset: Cultivate a positive attitude and practice gratitude. A positive outlook on life can boost overall well-being and immune function.

Avoid Overexertion:

Balanced Activities: Avoid excessive physical and mental strain, as overexertion can weaken the immune system.

Moderation in Technology Use:

Screen Time: Limit excessive screen time and practice digital detoxes to promote healthy sleep patterns.

Hygiene Practices:

Regular Showers: Maintain regular personal hygiene practices to prevent the buildup of harmful microorganisms on the skin.

Vaccination:

Vaccination Schedule: Stay up to date with recommended vaccinations to protect against preventable illnesses.

Mind-Body Practices:

Yoga and Tai Chi: Engage in mind-body practices like yoga and tai chi, which combine movement, breathing, and meditation to support immune function.

Maintaining a Healthy Weight:

Balanced Lifestyle: Adopt a balanced approach to diet and exercise to support a healthy weight, as excessive weight can impact immune function.

Limiting Exposure to Toxins:

Environmental Toxins: Minimize exposure to environmental toxins by choosing natural cleaning products, avoiding unnecessary chemicals, and reducing air pollution exposure.

Regular Medical Check-ups:

Health Assessments: Schedule regular medical check-ups and screenings to detect any underlying health issues.

Early Detection: Early detection and treatment of health conditions can prevent complications and support immune health.

Cultivating Resilience:

Adaptability: Develop coping skills to navigate challenges and build resilience against stressors.

Balancing Work and Rest:

Work-Life Balance: Prioritize a healthy work-life balance to avoid burnout and support overall well-being.

Hydration and Nutrition:

Water Intake: Stay hydrated by drinking an adequate amount of water throughout the day. Proper hydration supports immune system function and overall health.

Balanced Diet: Consume a well-balanced diet rich in fruits, vegetables, whole grains, lean proteins, and healthy fats. Nutrient intake is essential for immune cell production and function.

Emotional Well-Being:

Stress Reduction: Practice stress-relief techniques like deep breathing, meditation, journaling, or engaging in hobbies to maintain emotional well-being.

Positive Relationships: Foster positive relationships and social connections, which can contribute to mental and emotional resilience.

Moderate Alcohol Consumption:

Limitation: If you choose to drink alcohol, do so in moderation. Excessive alcohol consumption can suppress immune function.

Regular Physical Activity:

Regular Exercise: Engage in regular physical activity, which can boost circulation, enhance immune cell function, and reduce stress.

Outdoor Activities: Spend time outdoors and engage in activities like walking, jogging, hiking, or cycling for added benefits.

Proper Sleep Hygiene:

Consistent Sleep Schedule: Maintain a consistent sleep schedule by going to bed and waking up at the same times each day.

Sleep Environment: Create a comfortable sleep environment by keeping the room dark, quiet, and at a comfortable temperature.

Personal Hygiene:

Hand Hygiene: Wash hands frequently with soap and water, especially before eating or touching your face.

Oral Health: Maintain good oral hygiene by brushing and flossing regularly to prevent the entry of pathogens through the mouth.

Avoid Overexertion:

Balance: Engage in physical activities that challenge you without overexerting yourself. Rest and recovery are important for immune health.

Stay Informed:

Health Information: Stay informed about current health recommendations, vaccinations, and preventive measures to safeguard your immune health.

Mindfulness Practices:

Mindful Eating: Practice mindful eating, paying attention to your body's hunger and fullness cues.

Mindful Living: Apply mindfulness techniques to various aspects of your life to reduce stress and promote overall well-being.

Limit Processed Foods:

Whole Foods: Focus on whole, unprocessed foods rather than heavily processed and fast foods, which often lack essential nutrients.

Regular Medical Check-ups:

Health Assessments: Schedule regular check-ups with healthcare professionals to monitor your health status and catch potential issues early.

Environmental Factors:

Clean Environment: Maintain a clean and well-ventilated living and working environment to reduce exposure to pollutants and allergens.

Laughter and Joy:

Positive Emotions: Engage in activities that bring you joy and laughter. Positive emotions can contribute to overall well-being and immune function.

Personal Care:

Self-Care: Prioritize self-care activities such as relaxing baths, massages, and spending time doing things you love.

Limit Screen Time:

Digital Detox: Take breaks from electronic devices and screens to reduce eye strain and promote better sleep.

Adaptability:

Resilience: Develop the ability to adapt to changes and challenges. Resilience can positively impact overall health and immune function.

Gratitude and Positivity:

Gratitude Practice: Practice gratitude by focusing on positive aspects of your life. Gratitude can improve overall outlook and immune health.

Book 16: Restoring Digestive Health: Dr. Sebi's Remedies for a Happy Gut

Gut Health: Common Digestive Issues and Causes

Maintaining a healthy gut is essential for overall well-being. Digestive issues can impact various aspects of your health, from nutrient absorption to immune function. Understanding common digestive problems and their underlying causes is crucial for taking proactive steps to support your gut health. Here's a detailed explanation of some common digestive issues and their causes:

1. Acid Reflux (Gastroesophageal Reflux Disease- GERD):

- **Causes:** Acid reflux occurs when stomach acid flows back into the esophagus. Causes include a weakened lower esophageal sphincter (LES), obesity, pregnancy, certain foods (citrus, fatty foods, caffeine), and smoking.

2. Irritable Bowel Syndrome (IBS):

- **Causes:** The exact cause of IBS is unclear but may involve abnormal gut motility, visceral hypersensitivity, gut-brain communication issues, and changes in gut microbiota.

3. Inflammatory Bowel Disease (IBD)- Crohn's Disease and Ulcerative Colitis:

- **Causes:** These chronic conditions result from an overactive immune response against the gut, triggered by genetic and environmental factors.

4. Constipation:

- **Causes:** Constipation can result from low fiber intake, dehydration, lack of physical activity, medications, and certain medical conditions.

5. Diarrhea:

- **Causes:** Diarrhea may stem from infections, food intolerances, inflammatory conditions, medications, and digestive disorders like IBS.

6. Gallstones:

- **Causes:** Gallstones form when substances in bile (cholesterol, bilirubin) crystallize. They can cause pain and blockage in the bile ducts.

7. Celiac Disease:

- **Causes:** Celiac disease is an autoimmune disorder triggered by the consumption of gluten. The immune response damages the lining of the small intestine.

8. Diverticulitis:

- **Causes:** Diverticulitis involves inflammation or infection of small pouches (diverticula) in the colon. Causes may include low fiber intake and aging.

9. Gastroenteritis:

- **Causes:** Gastroenteritis, often called stomach flu, results from viral or bacterial infections that cause inflammation of the stomach and intestines.

10. Gastritis:

- **Causes:** Gastritis is inflammation of the stomach lining, often due to infection (H. pylori), alcohol consumption, certain medications, and stress.

11. Peptic Ulcers:

- **Causes:** Peptic ulcers are sores in the stomach, small intestine, or esophagus. H. pylori infection and use of nonsteroidal anti-inflammatory drugs (NSAIDs) are common causes.

12. Lactose Intolerance:

- **Causes:** Lactose intolerance occurs when the body lacks the enzyme lactase to digest lactose, the sugar in milk and dairy products.

13. Gastroesophageal Reflux Disease (GERD):

- **Causes:** GERD is a chronic condition where stomach acid frequently flows back into the esophagus. Causes include a weak LES, obesity, smoking, and certain foods.

14. Small Intestinal Bacterial Overgrowth (SIBO):

- **Causes:** SIBO occurs when there's an excessive growth of bacteria in the small intestine, leading to digestive symptoms.

15. Gastrointestinal Bleeding:

- **Causes:** Gastrointestinal bleeding can result from various factors, including ulcers, hemorrhoids, infections, and inflammatory conditions.

16. Dyspepsia (Indigestion):

- **Causes:** Indigestion can be caused by overeating, consuming fatty or spicy foods, stress, and certain medical conditions.

17. Food Allergies and Sensitivities:

- **Causes:** Food allergies and sensitivities can trigger digestive symptoms such as bloating, gas, diarrhea, and abdominal pain.

18. Excessive Gas:

- **Causes:** Gas can result from swallowing air, consuming gas-producing foods, and gut bacteria fermentation.

19. Gastroparesis:

- **Causes:** Gastroparesis is a condition where the stomach's emptying is delayed due to nerve or muscle dysfunction.

20. Eosinophilic Esophagitis:

- **Causes:** Eosinophilic esophagitis involves inflammation in the esophagus, often triggered by allergies to certain foods.

21. Gastrointestinal Motility Disorders:

- **Causes:** These disorders affect the movement of food through the digestive tract. They can result from nerve or muscle dysfunction, leading to symptoms like bloating, pain, and irregular bowel movements.

22. Gut Dysbiosis:

- **Causes:** An imbalance in the gut microbiota can lead to gut dysbiosis, potentially contributing to digestive problems and systemic health issues.

23. Malabsorption Syndromes:

- **Causes:** Conditions like celiac disease, Crohn's disease, and pancreatic insufficiency can impair nutrient absorption, leading to deficiencies and digestive symptoms.

24. Hemorrhoids:

- **Causes:** Hemorrhoids are swollen veins in the rectum or anus, often caused by straining during bowel movements, pregnancy, or prolonged sitting.

25. Cyclic Vomiting Syndrome:

- **Causes:** This condition involves recurring episodes of severe nausea, vomiting, and other gastrointestinal symptoms. The exact cause is unclear.

26. Gastric Outlet Obstruction:

- **Causes:** Gastric outlet obstruction occurs when the passage of food from the stomach to the small intestine is blocked, often due to a tumor or scar tissue.

27. Bowel Obstruction:

- **Causes:** Bowel obstruction can result from physical blockages, hernias, adhesions, or conditions like Crohn's disease.

28. Colorectal Cancer:

- **Causes:** Colorectal cancer develops when abnormal cells grow in the colon or rectum. Genetic and lifestyle factors contribute to its development.

29. Malnutrition:

- **Causes:** Digestive issues can lead to malnutrition due to inadequate nutrient absorption or increased nutrient losses.

30. Gut-Brain Axis Dysfunction:

- **Causes:** Dysregulation of the gut-brain axis can contribute to gastrointestinal symptoms and conditions like IBS and functional dyspepsia.

31. Autoimmune Diseases:

- **Causes:** Autoimmune diseases like autoimmune hepatitis and primary biliary cholangitis can affect the liver and bile ducts, leading to digestive symptoms.

32. Appendicitis:

- **Causes:** Appendicitis involves inflammation of the appendix, often due to obstruction of the appendix by stool or infection.

33. Biliary Colic:

- **Causes:** Biliary colic is caused by gallstones temporarily blocking the bile ducts, leading to intense pain.

34. Gastrointestinal Parasites:

- **Causes:** Infections by parasites like Giardia and Cryptosporidium can lead to digestive symptoms like diarrhea and abdominal pain.

35. Pancreatitis:

- **Causes:** Pancreatitis is inflammation of the pancreas, often linked to alcohol consumption, gallstones, and certain medications.

36. FODMAP Sensitivity:

- **Causes:** Some individuals are sensitive to certain fermentable carbohydrates (FODMAPs), leading to digestive symptoms like bloating and diarrhea.

37. Gut Permeability (Leaky Gut):

- **Causes:** Increased gut permeability can result from factors like chronic inflammation, poor diet, and imbalanced gut microbiota.

38. Exocrine Pancreatic Insufficiency (EPI):

- **Causes:** EPI occurs when the pancreas doesn't produce enough digestive enzymes, impairing nutrient absorption.

39. Functional Gastrointestinal Disorders:

- **Causes:** Conditions like functional dyspepsia, functional diarrhea, and functional constipation involve abnormal gut function without structural abnormalities.

40. Overeating and Poor Eating Habits:

- **Causes:** Overeating, eating too quickly, and consuming excessive fatty or processed foods can lead to digestive discomfort and issues.

Dr. Sebi's Herbal Support for Digestive Health

Dr. Sebi, a natural healer and herbalist, believed in using natural herbs to promote overall health and wellness, including digestive health. While I can provide some general information about Dr. Sebi's herbal recommendations, please note that individual responses to herbs can vary, and it's important to consult with a healthcare professional before incorporating new herbs into your routine. Here are some herbs that Dr. Sebi commonly recommended for supporting digestive health:

1. Aloe Vera:

- **Benefits:** Aloe vera is known for its soothing properties and potential to help with digestive discomfort and inflammation.

2. Burdock Root:

- **Benefits:** Burdock root is believed to support digestion by promoting detoxification and aiding in the elimination of waste from the body.

3. Dandelion:

- **Benefits:** Dandelion is thought to stimulate digestion and support liver function, which plays a key role in detoxification.

4. Chaparral:

- **Benefits:** Chaparral has been used traditionally to aid digestion and address gastrointestinal issues.

5. Sarsaparilla:

- **Benefits:** Sarsaparilla is believed to have anti-inflammatory properties and may contribute to overall digestive well-being.

6. Yellow Dock:

- **Benefits:** Yellow dock is often used to support liver health, which is crucial for efficient digestion and toxin elimination.

7. Irish Moss:

- **Benefits:** Irish moss is rich in minerals and may have soothing properties for the digestive tract.

8. Bromide Plus Powder:

- **Benefits:** This herbal blend is intended to support healthy bowel movements and overall gut health.

9. Bladderwrack:

- **Benefits:** Bladderwrack is thought to promote healthy digestion and support thyroid function, which can influence metabolism.

10. Seamoss:

- **Benefits:** Seamoss, also known as Irish moss, is believed to have a mucilaginous quality that can soothe and support the digestive tract.

11. Cascara Sagrada:

- **Benefits:** Cascara sagrada is traditionally used as a natural laxative to promote regular bowel movements.

12. Burdock Root:

- **Benefits:** Burdock root may help stimulate digestion, support liver health, and aid in detoxification.

13. Senna Leaf:

- **Benefits:** Senna leaf is sometimes used for its natural laxative properties to support bowel regularity.

14. Cascara Sagrada:

- **Benefits:** Cascara sagrada is a natural laxative that can help support bowel movements and relieve constipation.

15. African Bird Pepper:

- **Benefits:** African bird pepper is believed to have digestive benefits and may help stimulate metabolism.

16. Chaparral:

- **Benefits:** Chaparral has been traditionally used to support digestion and address gastrointestinal issues.

17. Sarsaparilla:

- **Benefits:** Sarsaparilla is thought to have anti-inflammatory properties that can potentially benefit digestion.

18. Bromide Plus Powder:

- **Benefits:** This herbal blend is designed to support bowel health and contribute to overall digestive wellness.

19. Bitter Melon:

- **Benefits:** Bitter melon is believed to have digestive benefits and may help regulate blood sugar levels.

20. Cocolmeca:

- **Benefits:** Cocolmeca is used in traditional medicine for digestive support and overall wellness.

21. Sage:

- **Benefits:** Sage is believed to have antimicrobial properties and may aid in digestion by promoting a healthy balance of gut bacteria.

22. Bitter Herbs (Gentian, Wormwood, Mugwort):

- **Benefits:** Bitter herbs are thought to stimulate digestive enzymes, improve appetite, and support the overall digestive process.

23. Ginger:

- **Benefits:** Ginger is known for its anti-inflammatory and soothing properties, which can help alleviate digestive discomfort and promote healthy digestion.

24. Peppermint:

- **Benefits:** Peppermint is often used to relieve symptoms of indigestion, such as bloating and gas.

25. Fennel:

- **Benefits:** Fennel seeds are believed to support digestion by reducing bloating, cramping, and indigestion.

26. Licorice Root:

- **Benefits:** Licorice root is thought to have anti-inflammatory properties that may help soothe the digestive tract.

27. Plantain Leaf:

- **Benefits:** Plantain leaf is believed to support gastrointestinal health by promoting healing and reducing inflammation.

28. Mullein Leaf:

- **Benefits:** Mullein leaf is traditionally used to soothe mucous membranes and support respiratory and digestive health.

29. Chickweed:

- **Benefits:** Chickweed is thought to have anti-inflammatory and soothing properties that can support digestive comfort.

30. Red Clover:

- **Benefits:** Red clover is often used for detoxification and supporting overall digestive wellness.

31. Golden Seal:

- **Benefits:** Golden seal is believed to have antimicrobial properties and may help support digestion and immune health.

32. Black Walnut Hull:

- **Benefits:** Black walnut hull is used for its potential to support digestive health and promote detoxification.

33. Nettle:

- **Benefits:** Nettle is rich in nutrients and may contribute to overall digestive and immune system support.

34. Moringa:

- **Benefits:** Moringa is nutrient-dense and believed to have anti-inflammatory properties that can contribute to digestive well-being.

35. Sage:

- **Benefits:** Sage is known for its antimicrobial properties and potential to support healthy gut flora.

36. Marshmallow Root:

- **Benefits:** Marshmallow root is used for its mucilaginous quality, which can soothe the digestive tract and promote healing.

37. Agrimony:

- **Benefits:** Agrimony is believed to support digestion and alleviate gastrointestinal discomfort.

38. Yarrow:

- **Benefits:** Yarrow is traditionally used to support digestion and promote overall well-being.

39. Rosemary:

- **Benefits:** Rosemary is thought to stimulate digestion and may have antioxidant properties that support gut health.

40. Calendula:

- **Benefits:** Calendula is believed to have anti-inflammatory properties that can benefit digestive comfort.

The Alkaline Diet for a Balanced Gut

The alkaline diet is based on the principle that consuming certain foods can help maintain a balanced pH level in the body, which in turn can support overall health, including gut health. While the alkaline diet has gained popularity, it's important to note that the body's pH regulation is complex, and the impact of dietary pH on gut health may not be as straightforward as suggested. However, the alkaline diet does emphasize consumption of nutrient-rich whole foods that can contribute to gut well-being. Here's a detailed explanation of the alkaline diet's potential benefits for a balanced gut:

1. Fruits and Vegetables:

- **Benefits:** Many fruits and vegetables are alkaline-forming, providing essential vitamins, minerals, antioxidants, and dietary fiber that support gut health. Fiber promotes regular bowel movements and feeds beneficial gut bacteria.

2. Leafy Greens:

- **Benefits:** Leafy greens like kale, spinach, and Swiss chard are highly alkaline and rich in vitamins, minerals, and phytonutrients that promote gut wellness.

3. Cruciferous Vegetables:

- **Benefits:** Cruciferous vegetables such as broccoli, cauliflower, and Brussels sprouts are alkaline-forming and contain compounds that may support digestion and detoxification.

4. Berries:

- **Benefits:** Berries like blueberries, strawberries, and raspberries are low in sugar and rich in antioxidants that may contribute to a diverse and balanced gut microbiome.

5. Nuts and Seeds:

- **Benefits:** Almonds, walnuts, and flaxseeds are alkaline-forming and provide healthy fats, fiber, and nutrients that can support gut health.

6. Legumes:

- **Benefits:** Beans, lentils, and chickpeas are rich in fiber, protein, and prebiotics that nourish beneficial gut bacteria.

7. Whole Grains:

- **Benefits:** Quinoa, brown rice, and oats can contribute to a balanced gut by providing fiber and nutrients that support digestion.

8. Healthy Fats:

- **Benefits:** Avocado, olive oil, and coconut oil are considered alkaline-forming and provide beneficial fats that can support a healthy gut lining.

9. Herbs and Spices:

- **Benefits:** Many herbs and spices like turmeric, ginger, and garlic have anti-inflammatory and digestive benefits that can contribute to gut wellness.

10. Plant-Based Proteins:

- **Benefits:** Plant-based proteins like tofu and tempeh are alkaline-forming and can be part of a balanced diet that supports gut health.

11. Hydration:

- **Benefits:** Staying hydrated with water and herbal teas supports digestion, nutrient absorption, and the elimination of waste.

12. Reduced Processed Foods and Sugar:

- **Benefits:** The alkaline diet encourages reducing processed foods and sugar, which can contribute to a more diverse and balanced gut microbiome.

13. Limited Animal Products:

- **Benefits:** While the alkaline diet suggests limited animal products, plant-based options can provide similar nutrients while also supporting gut health through fiber and antioxidants.

14. pH Balance and Gut Health:

- **Benefits:** While the body naturally maintains its own pH balance, consuming alkaline-forming foods can provide a variety of nutrients that contribute to gut wellness.

15. Prebiotic-Rich Foods:

- **Benefits:** Foods rich in prebiotics, such as garlic, onions, leeks, asparagus, and bananas, nourish beneficial gut bacteria and promote a balanced gut microbiome.

16. Fermented Foods:

- **Benefits:** Incorporating fermented foods like sauerkraut, kimchi, kefir, and yogurt can introduce probiotics to the gut, supporting microbial diversity and digestion.

17. Alkaline Water:

- **Benefits:** Alkaline water is promoted in the alkaline diet for its potential to help balance pH levels. However, scientific evidence supporting its impact on gut health is limited.

18. Herbal Teas:

- **Benefits:** Herbal teas like chamomile, peppermint, and ginger can have soothing effects on the digestive system, promoting comfort and relaxation.

19. Anti-Inflammatory Effects:

- **Benefits:** Many alkaline-forming foods, such as leafy greens and berries, have anti-inflammatory properties that can contribute to a healthier gut environment.

20. Gut Barrier Integrity:

- **Benefits:** The alkaline diet's emphasis on whole foods, especially plant-based options, can support the integrity of the gut barrier, preventing leaky gut and inflammation.

21. Reduced Acidic Foods:

- **Benefits:** The alkaline diet suggests limiting acidic foods like processed meats, refined sugars, and high-sugar beverages, which may contribute to gut inflammation.

22. Plant Diversity:

- **Benefits:** Consuming a wide variety of alkaline-forming plant foods can promote a diverse gut microbiome, which is associated with better gut health.

23. Reduced Inflammation:

- **Benefits:** The alkaline diet's focus on anti-inflammatory foods can potentially reduce gut inflammation, improving overall gut function.

24. Gut-Brain Connection:

- **Benefits:** Some alkaline-forming foods, such as leafy greens and fatty fish, may support the gut-brain axis, influencing mood and gut health.

25. Whole Food Nutrients:

- **Benefits:** Alkaline-forming whole foods provide essential nutrients like vitamins, minerals, and antioxidants that support gut health and overall well-being.

26. Balanced Microbiome:

- **Benefits:** The combination of fiber-rich foods and prebiotic-rich options in the alkaline diet can promote a balanced and thriving gut microbiome.

27. Improved Digestion:

- **Benefits:** Alkaline-forming foods like fruits, vegetables, and whole grains provide dietary fiber that supports regular bowel movements and efficient digestion.

28. Maintained Weight:

- **Benefits:** Following the alkaline diet's emphasis on whole foods and reducing processed options can contribute to a healthy weight, which supports gut health.

Conclusion:

While the alkaline diet's direct impact on gut pH may be debated, its focus on nutrient-dense, alkaline-forming foods aligns with principles that support a balanced gut microbiome and overall digestive well-being. Remember that individual responses to the diet can vary, and it's important to consult with a healthcare professional before making significant dietary changes. Combining the alkaline diet's principles with other factors such as regular exercise, stress management, and proper sleep can contribute to optimal gut health and a healthier lifestyle.

Lifestyle Practices for Digestive Wellness

In addition to dietary choices, lifestyle practices play a crucial role in maintaining digestive wellness. Adopting healthy habits can support optimal digestion, gut health, and overall well-being. Here are detailed explanations of lifestyle practices that can contribute to digestive wellness:

1. Mindful Eating:

- **Benefits:** Practicing mindful eating involves paying full attention to your meal, savoring each bite, and eating slowly. This practice helps signal to your body when you're full and supports proper digestion.

2. Hydration:

- **Benefits:** Staying hydrated is essential for digestion, as water helps break down food and supports the absorption of nutrients. Aim to drink adequate water throughout the day.

3. Regular Exercise:

- **Benefits:** Engaging in regular physical activity can promote healthy digestion by encouraging the movement of food through the digestive tract and reducing the risk of constipation.

4. Stress Management:

- **Benefits:** Chronic stress can impact digestion by altering gut motility and increasing inflammation. Practices such as meditation, deep breathing, and yoga can help manage stress and support gut health.

5. Adequate Sleep:

- **Benefits:** Getting enough sleep is crucial for proper digestion and overall health. Poor sleep can disrupt digestion and lead to issues like indigestion and bloating.

6. Chewing Thoroughly:

- **Benefits:** Properly chewing your food breaks it down into smaller particles, making it easier for enzymes to work and aiding in the digestion process.

7. Regular Meals and Snacking:

- **Benefits:** Eating regular meals and balanced snacks helps regulate blood sugar levels and maintains a steady release of digestive enzymes.

8. Fiber-Rich Diet:

- **Benefits:** Consuming sufficient dietary fiber supports healthy bowel movements and provides prebiotics that nourish beneficial gut bacteria.

9. Limiting Processed Foods:

- **Benefits:** Processed foods are often low in nutrients and high in unhealthy fats and sugars. Reducing their consumption can promote a healthier gut and overall well-being.

10. Limiting Alcohol and Caffeine:

- **Benefits:** Excessive alcohol and caffeine consumption can irritate the digestive tract and disrupt gut health. Moderation is key.

11. Avoiding Overeating:

- **Benefits:** Overeating can overwhelm the digestive system, leading to discomfort, indigestion, and bloating. Eating until you're comfortably satisfied is ideal.

12. Meal Timing:

- **Benefits:** Consistent meal times help regulate digestion and promote efficient nutrient absorption.

13. Probiotics and Prebiotics:

- **Benefits:** Incorporating foods rich in probiotics (fermented foods) and prebiotics (fiber-rich foods) can support a balanced gut microbiome.

Book 17: Beating Insomnia Naturally: Dr. Sebi's Guide to Restful Sleep

Understanding Insomnia: Causes and Symptoms

Insomnia is a common sleep disorder characterized by difficulty falling asleep, staying asleep, or experiencing non-restorative sleep, despite having the opportunity to do so. It can have a significant impact on an individual's overall well-being, affecting their mood, energy levels, and daily functioning. Here's a detailed explanation of the causes and symptoms of insomnia:

Causes of Insomnia:

Stress and Anxiety:

- **Explanation:** Stressful life events, work pressures, and personal worries can lead to racing thoughts and increased arousal, making it difficult to relax and fall asleep.

Poor Sleep Hygiene:

- **Explanation:** Irregular sleep schedules, excessive daytime napping, and inconsistent bedtime routines can disrupt the body's natural sleep-wake cycle, contributing to insomnia.

Medical Conditions:

- **Explanation:** Certain medical conditions such as chronic pain, allergies, asthma, acid reflux, and hormonal imbalances can cause discomfort and disrupt sleep.

Mental Health Disorders:

- **Explanation:** Conditions like depression, anxiety, and post-traumatic stress disorder (PTSD) can interfere with sleep patterns and lead to insomnia.

Medications:

- **Explanation:** Some medications, such as certain antidepressants, stimulants, and medications for asthma or high blood pressure, can interfere with sleep.

Caffeine and Alcohol Consumption:

- **Explanation:** Consuming caffeine or alcohol close to bedtime can disrupt sleep by affecting the body's ability to enter deeper sleep stages.

Environmental Factors:

- **Explanation:** Noise, light, an uncomfortable mattress, and a disruptive sleep environment can all contribute to difficulty falling and staying asleep.

Shift Work or Jet Lag:

- **Explanation:** Disruptions to the body's internal clock due to irregular work hours or travel across time zones can lead to sleep disturbances.

Symptoms of Insomnia:

Difficulty Falling Asleep:

- **Explanation:** Individuals with insomnia may experience prolonged periods of lying in bed unable to fall asleep, even when they feel tired.

Frequent Waking at Night:

- **Explanation:** Insomnia can cause individuals to wake up multiple times during the night, often struggling to return to sleep.

Non-Restorative Sleep:

- **Explanation:** Even after getting sleep, individuals with insomnia may wake up feeling unrefreshed and fatigued, impacting their daytime functioning.

Daytime Sleepiness:

- **Explanation:** Insomnia can lead to excessive daytime sleepiness, reduced alertness, and difficulty concentrating, affecting work or daily activities.

Mood Disturbances:

- **Explanation:** Insomnia is associated with mood changes such as irritability, mood swings, and an increased risk of developing mood disorders.

Difficulty Concentrating:

- **Explanation:** Sleep deprivation caused by insomnia can impair cognitive functions, making it challenging to focus, make decisions, or remember things.

Physical Symptoms:

- **Explanation:** Insomnia can lead to physical symptoms such as headaches, muscle tension, and gastrointestinal distress.

Dependency on Sleep Aids:

- **Explanation:** In an attempt to manage insomnia, individuals may develop a reliance on sleep medications or substances like alcohol.

Coping with Insomnia: Strategies for Better Sleep

Coping with insomnia involves adopting various strategies to improve sleep quality and establish healthy sleep habits. By making positive changes to your daily routine and environment, you can effectively manage insomnia and promote restful sleep. Here's a detailed exploration of strategies for better sleep:

Sleep Hygiene:

Explanation: Establish a consistent sleep schedule by going to bed and waking up at the same times every day, even on weekends. This helps regulate your body's internal clock.

Create a Relaxing Bedtime Routine:

Explanation: Engage in calming activities before bed, such as reading, taking a warm bath, practicing relaxation techniques, or gentle yoga.

Limit Screen Time:

Explanation: Avoid electronic devices with screens (phones, tablets, computers) at least an hour before bedtime. The blue light emitted by screens can interfere with the production of the sleep-inducing hormone melatonin.

Comfortable Sleep Environment:

Explanation: Ensure your bedroom is conducive to sleep by keeping it cool, dark, and quiet. Invest in a comfortable mattress and pillows to support restful sleep.

Manage Stress and Anxiety:

Explanation: Practice stress reduction techniques such as deep breathing, meditation, or mindfulness to calm your mind before bed.

Limit Caffeine and Alcohol:

Explanation: Avoid consuming caffeine or alcohol close to bedtime, as they can disrupt sleep patterns and quality.

Be Mindful of Food Choices:

Explanation: Avoid heavy meals and spicy foods before bed, as they can cause discomfort and acid reflux.

Physical Activity:

Explanation: Engage in regular physical activity, but avoid intense exercise close to bedtime. Aim for physical activity earlier in the day to promote better sleep.

Limit Naps:

Explanation: If you nap during the day, keep it short (20-30 minutes) and avoid napping too close to bedtime, as it can interfere with nighttime sleep.

Avoid Clock-Watching:

Explanation: If you have trouble falling asleep, avoid constantly checking the clock, as this can increase anxiety and make it harder to relax.

Cognitive Behavioral Therapy for Insomnia (CBT-I):

Explanation: CBT-I is a structured program that helps individuals identify and change negative thought patterns and behaviors associated with sleep. It's an effective long-term solution for managing insomnia.

Natural Remedies:

Explanation: Herbal teas such as chamomile, valerian, or lavender can have calming effects and promote relaxation before bedtime.

White Noise or Relaxing Sounds:

Explanation: Using white noise machines, calming music, or nature sounds can create a soothing environment that promotes better sleep.

Establish a Wind-Down Routine:

Explanation: Gradually wind down your activities in the evening, creating a buffer between stimulating activities and sleep.

Seek Professional Help:

Explanation: If insomnia persists despite trying these strategies, consult a healthcare professional. They can provide personalized guidance and recommendations based on your individual situation.

Dr. Sebi's Herbal Recommendations for Better Sleep

Dr. Sebi was a Honduran herbalist and advocate for natural healing who believed that consuming a plant-based, alkaline-rich diet and using specific herbs could contribute to overall well-being, including improved sleep quality. While individual responses to herbs may vary, Dr. Sebi's approach to herbal remedies aimed to support the body's natural healing processes. Here are some of Dr. Sebi's herbal recommendations that may contribute to better sleep:

1. Valerian Root (Valeriana officinalis):

- **Explanation:** Valerian root has been traditionally used for its calming and sedative effects, which may help ease anxiety and promote relaxation, leading to better sleep.

2. Chamomile (Matricaria chamomilla):

- **Explanation:** Chamomile is known for its soothing properties. It can be consumed as a tea and may help relax the mind and body before bedtime.

3. Passionflower (Passiflora incarnata):

- **Explanation:** Passionflower is often used to alleviate anxiety and promote relaxation. It may help reduce racing thoughts and support a calm state conducive to sleep.

4. Lavender (Lavandula angustifolia):

- **Explanation:** Lavender is renowned for its calming aroma. It can be used as an essential oil, added to a bath, or inhaled before bedtime to induce relaxation.

5. Skullcap (Scutellaria lateriflora):

- **Explanation:** Skullcap has been used as a nerve tonic and relaxant. It may help soothe nervous tension and contribute to better sleep.

6. California Poppy (Eschscholzia californica):

- **Explanation:** California poppy is often used for its mild sedative properties. It may help ease anxiety and nervousness, promoting a more peaceful sleep.

7. Hops (Humulus lupulus):

- **Explanation:** Hops are commonly associated with their use in beer-making, but they also have mild sedative effects that can contribute to relaxation and improved sleep quality.

8. Lemon Balm (Melissa officinalis):

- **Explanation:** Lemon balm is known for its calming effects and is used to alleviate stress and anxiety. It can be consumed as a tea before bedtime.

9. Wild Lettuce (Lactuca virosa):

- **Explanation:** Wild lettuce is believed to have sedative properties that may help relax the body and mind, potentially leading to better sleep.

10. Ashwagandha (Withania somnifera):

- **Explanation:** Ashwagandha is an adaptogenic herb that may help reduce stress and support the body's ability to adapt to various stressors, potentially leading to improved sleep.

11. Ginger (Zingiber officinale):

- **Explanation:** Ginger is often used for its anti-inflammatory properties. Consuming ginger tea or incorporating it into your diet may contribute to overall well-being, which can indirectly support better sleep.

12. Kava Kava (Piper methysticum):

- **Explanation:** Kava kava has been used in some cultures for its calming effects. It's important to use kava kava cautiously and under the guidance of a healthcare professional, as it may interact with other medications.

Note: Before incorporating any herbal remedies, including those suggested by Dr. Sebi, it's essential to consult with a qualified healthcare professional, especially if you have existing medical conditions, are taking medications, or are pregnant or nursing. Herbal remedies can have individual variations in effectiveness and potential interactions, so it's important to ensure they are safe and suitable for your specific health circumstances.

The Alkaline Diet for Restful Sleep

The alkaline diet, popularized by Dr. Sebi, emphasizes consuming foods that are considered alkaline-forming in the body. While there is limited scientific evidence directly linking the alkaline diet to improved sleep, a diet rich in nutrient-dense, plant-based foods can positively impact overall well-being, which may indirectly contribute to better sleep quality. Here's an exploration of how the alkaline diet can potentially support restful sleep:

1. Plant-Based Foods:

- **Explanation:** The alkaline diet encourages consuming a variety of plant-based foods, such as vegetables, fruits, nuts, seeds, and whole grains. These foods are rich in vitamins, minerals, and antioxidants that support overall health, which can indirectly promote better sleep.

2. Hydration:

- **Explanation:** The alkaline diet emphasizes staying hydrated by consuming water and hydrating foods like cucumbers and watermelon. Adequate hydration supports various bodily functions, including maintaining healthy sleep patterns.

3. Mineral-Rich Foods:

- **Explanation:** The diet promotes foods that are rich in alkaline minerals like magnesium and potassium, which play roles in muscle relaxation, nervous system function, and sleep regulation.

4. Reduced Acidic Foods:

- **Explanation:** The alkaline diet encourages reducing consumption of highly acidic foods, such as processed foods, sugar, and excessive animal products. High-acid diets may contribute to inflammation and discomfort that can interfere with sleep.

5. Omega-3 Fatty Acids:

- **Explanation:** Incorporating plant-based sources of omega-3 fatty acids, like flaxseeds, chia seeds, and walnuts, may support brain health and overall well-being, potentially benefiting sleep quality.

6. Balanced Blood Sugar Levels:

- **Explanation:** The diet's emphasis on whole, unprocessed foods with a low glycemic index can help regulate blood sugar levels. Stable blood sugar levels contribute to more consistent energy levels and better sleep patterns.

7. Fiber Intake:

- **Explanation:** Plant-based foods are often high in dietary fiber, which supports healthy digestion. Good digestion can reduce discomfort and disruptions that might otherwise interfere with sleep.

8. Antioxidant-Rich Foods:

- **Explanation:** Alkaline foods are often rich in antioxidants that combat oxidative stress. Reduced oxidative stress can positively impact overall health, including potential benefits for sleep.

9. Mindful Eating:

- **Explanation:** Following an alkaline diet encourages mindful eating and awareness of the foods you consume. This can promote a healthier relationship with food, stress reduction, and relaxation.

10. Reduced Caffeine and Sugar:

- **Explanation:** An alkaline diet discourages excessive consumption of caffeine and refined sugars, both of which can disrupt sleep patterns and quality.

11. Limiting Processed Foods:

- **Explanation:** The alkaline diet encourages choosing whole, natural foods over processed and refined options, which can support general health and vitality, potentially leading to better sleep.

Lifestyle Habits for Promoting Restful Sleep

Creating healthy lifestyle habits is crucial for fostering restful sleep. These habits contribute to improved sleep quality by creating a conducive environment for relaxation and sleep. By integrating these practices into your daily routine, you can establish a foundation for better sleep and overall well-being. Here's an in-depth exploration of lifestyle habits that promote restful sleep:

1. Consistent Sleep Schedule:

- **Explanation:** Go to bed and wake up at the same time every day, even on weekends. Consistency helps regulate your body's internal clock, making it easier to fall asleep and wake up naturally.

2. Create a Relaxing Bedtime Routine:

- **Explanation:** Develop a calming pre-sleep routine that includes activities like reading, taking a warm bath, practicing relaxation techniques, or gentle stretching.

3. Limit Screen Time Before Bed:

- **Explanation:** Reduce exposure to electronic devices with screens (phones, tablets, computers) at least an hour before bedtime. Blue light emitted by screens can interfere with the production of melatonin, a sleep-inducing hormone.

4. Optimize Sleep Environment:

- **Explanation:** Make your bedroom conducive to sleep by keeping it cool, dark, and quiet. Invest in a comfortable mattress and pillows that support your sleeping posture.

5. Engage in Regular Exercise:

- **Explanation:** Engaging in regular physical activity can improve sleep quality. Aim for at least 30 minutes of moderate exercise most days, but avoid intense workouts close to bedtime.

6. Practice Relaxation Techniques:

- **Explanation:** Incorporate relaxation practices such as deep breathing, meditation, or progressive muscle relaxation before bed to calm your mind and prepare your body for sleep.

7. Limit Caffeine and Alcohol:

- **Explanation:** Avoid consuming caffeine and alcohol close to bedtime, as they can disrupt sleep patterns and affect sleep quality.

8. Stress Management:

- **Explanation:** Engage in stress-reducing activities like mindfulness, yoga, or journaling to alleviate stress and create a more relaxed mental state before bedtime.

9. Balanced Nutrition and Hydration:

- **Explanation:** Consume balanced meals and stay hydrated throughout the day. Avoid heavy meals and excessive fluids close to bedtime to prevent disruptions.

10. Wind Down Before Bed:

- **Explanation:** Engage in calming activities such as reading, listening to soothing music, or practicing gentle stretches to signal to your body that it's time to relax.

11. Unplug from Devices:

- **Explanation:** Reduce exposure to screens before bedtime. The blue light emitted by screens can suppress melatonin production and hinder sleep.

12. Avoid Heavy Meals Before Bed:

- **Explanation:** Refrain from consuming large, heavy meals close to bedtime. Indigestion and discomfort can disrupt your sleep.

13. Establish a Bedtime Routine:

- **Explanation:** Create a consistent routine that signals to your body that it's time to wind down. This can include activities like dimming lights, reading, or practicing relaxation exercises.

14. Stay Mindful of Napping:

- **Explanation:** If you need to nap during the day, keep it short and avoid napping too close to bedtime to prevent interference with nighttime sleep.

15. Create a Relaxing Atmosphere:

- **Explanation:** Make your bedroom a comfortable and peaceful space. Adjust lighting, temperature, and noise levels to your preference.

Book 18: Mental Clarity Unleashed: Dr. Sebi's Path to Cognitive Health

Cognitive Health: Enhancing Memory and Focus

Cognitive health is essential for maintaining optimal brain function, memory, and focus throughout your life. By adopting certain lifestyle practices and incorporating brain-boosting activities, you can enhance your cognitive abilities and support your brain's overall well-being. Here's an in-depth exploration of how to enhance memory and focus for better cognitive health:

1. Nutrition for Brain Health:

- **Explanation:** A balanced diet rich in nutrients is crucial for cognitive function. Foods rich in antioxidants, omega-3 fatty acids, vitamins, and minerals support brain health. Examples include leafy greens, fatty fish, berries, nuts, and whole grains.

2. Hydration for Brain Function:

- **Explanation:** Staying hydrated is essential for optimal brain function. Dehydration can lead to cognitive deficits, so drink enough water throughout the day.

3. Regular Physical Activity:

- **Explanation:** Engaging in regular exercise improves blood flow to the brain, promoting the growth of new neurons and enhancing cognitive function. Aim for a mix of cardiovascular and strength exercises.

4. Quality Sleep:

- **Explanation:** Prioritize getting adequate and restful sleep. Sleep is essential for memory consolidation and cognitive restoration.

5. Mindful Stress Management:

- **Explanation:** Chronic stress can negatively impact cognitive function. Practice stress-reduction techniques such as meditation, deep breathing, and mindfulness to promote mental clarity.

6. Brain-Boosting Activities:

- **Explanation:** Engage in activities that challenge your brain, such as puzzles, crosswords, Sudoku, and memory games. These activities stimulate neural connections and enhance cognitive abilities.

7. Social Engagement:

- **Explanation:** Maintaining social connections and engaging in meaningful interactions supports cognitive health. Social engagement stimulates brain activity and may reduce the risk of cognitive decline.

8. Learning and Lifelong Education:

- **Explanation:** Continuously seek opportunities for learning and personal growth. Engage in hobbies, take courses, or learn new skills to keep your brain active and adaptable.

9. Mindful Technology Use:

- **Explanation:** While technology can be beneficial, excessive screen time can impact cognitive health. Set limits on screen use and engage in activities that foster real-world connections.

10. Regular Mental Breaks:

- **Explanation:** Give your brain regular breaks throughout the day. Short breaks can improve focus and prevent mental fatigue.

11. Stay Hydrated:

- **Explanation:** Dehydration can impair cognitive function. Aim to drink enough water to stay hydrated, as even mild dehydration can affect memory and focus.

12. Limit Sugar and Processed Foods:

- **Explanation:** A diet high in sugar and processed foods may contribute to cognitive decline. Opt for whole foods and minimize sugary and processed snacks.

13. Brain-Boosting Supplements:

- **Explanation:** Consult with a healthcare professional before considering any supplements that claim to enhance cognitive function. Some supplements, like omega-3 fatty acids and certain vitamins, may support brain health.

14. Regular Cognitive Assessments:

- **Explanation:** Consider engaging in cognitive assessments or brain training apps that help track your cognitive performance over time.

15. Manage Chronic Conditions:

- **Explanation:** If you have underlying health conditions like diabetes or hypertension, manage them effectively, as they can impact cognitive health.

Dr. Sebi's Herbal Remedies for Brain Health

Dr. Sebi's herbal recommendations for brain health align with his holistic approach to overall well-being. While it's important to note that individual responses to herbs can vary, Dr. Sebi's suggestions emphasize nourishing and supporting the body's natural processes. Here's a detailed exploration of some of the herbs he recommended for brain health:

1. Ginkgo Biloba:

- **Explanation:** Ginkgo biloba is a well-known herb used to support cognitive function and enhance memory. It's believed to improve blood flow to the brain, which can promote optimal brain function and memory recall.

2. Gotu Kola:

- **Explanation:** Gotu kola is often used in traditional herbal medicine to enhance brain health. It's believed to support mental clarity, concentration, and overall cognitive function.

3. Sage:

- **Explanation:** Sage is rich in antioxidants and compounds that have been associated with improved memory and cognitive function. It may support brain health by protecting against oxidative stress.

4. Rosemary:

- **Explanation:** Rosemary contains compounds that have been shown to enhance cognitive performance and memory. Its aromatic properties are believed to have a positive impact on mental clarity.

5. Brahmi (Bacopa Monnieri):

- **Explanation:** Brahmi is an Ayurvedic herb known for its potential to enhance memory, learning, and cognitive function. It's believed to support neurotransmitter balance in the brain.

6. Ashwagandha:

- **Explanation:** Ashwagandha is an adaptogenic herb that helps the body manage stress. By reducing stress levels, it indirectly supports cognitive health and mental clarity.

7. Turmeric:

- **Explanation:** Turmeric contains curcumin, a compound with potent anti-inflammatory and antioxidant properties. It may protect the brain from inflammation and oxidative stress.

8. Lion's Mane Mushroom:

- **Explanation:** Lion's mane mushroom has gained attention for its potential to support brain health. It may stimulate the growth of nerve cells and enhance cognitive function.

9. Moringa:

- **Explanation:** Moringa is a nutrient-dense herb rich in vitamins, minerals, and antioxidants. Its nutritional profile may indirectly support brain health and overall well-being.

10. Black Seed (Nigella Sativa):

- **Explanation:** Black seed, also known as Nigella sativa, has been studied for its potential neuroprotective properties. It contains compounds that may support brain health and cognitive function.

11. Nettle Leaf:

- **Explanation:** Nettle leaf is a nutrient-rich herb that may contribute to overall health and well-being. Its vitamins and minerals can indirectly support brain function.

12. Mucuna Pruriens:

- **Explanation:** Mucuna pruriens contains L-DOPA, a precursor to dopamine, a neurotransmitter associated with mood and cognitive function. It may support mental clarity and well-being.

13. Oat Straw (Avena Sativa):

- **Explanation:** Oat straw is believed to have calming and soothing effects on the nervous system. It may indirectly support cognitive function by promoting relaxation.

14. Yerba Mate:

- **Explanation:** Yerba mate contains caffeine and compounds that can enhance alertness and mental clarity. It may provide a natural boost to cognitive function.

15. Schisandra Berry:

- **Explanation:** Schisandra berry is an adaptogenic herb that may help the body manage stress. By reducing stress, it indirectly supports brain health and cognitive function.

The Alkaline Diet for Cognitive Enhancement

The alkaline diet focuses on consuming foods that promote an alkaline environment in the body, which proponents believe can contribute to overall health, including cognitive enhancement. While scientific research on the direct impact of the alkaline diet on cognitive function is limited, the diet's emphasis on nutrient-rich, plant-based foods aligns with principles that support brain health. Here's an in-depth exploration of how the alkaline diet can be beneficial for cognitive enhancement:

1. Plant-Based Foods:

- **Explanation:** The alkaline diet encourages a high intake of plant-based foods, such as vegetables, fruits, legumes, nuts, and seeds. These foods are rich in antioxidants, vitamins, and minerals that support brain health and protect against oxidative stress.

2. Leafy Greens:

- **Explanation:** Leafy greens like spinach, kale, and Swiss chard are highly alkaline and contain nutrients like folate and vitamin K, which are important for cognitive function and brain health.

3. Healthy Fats:

- **Explanation:** The diet promotes healthy fats from sources like avocados, nuts, and seeds. Omega-3 fatty acids, found in foods like flaxseeds and walnuts, are associated with improved cognitive function and may support brain health.

4. Low Processed Foods:

- **Explanation:** The alkaline diet discourages highly processed and refined foods. This helps reduce the consumption of added sugars, unhealthy fats, and artificial additives that can negatively impact cognitive function.

5. Reduced Sugar Intake:

- **Explanation:** The diet's focus on whole foods can naturally lead to reduced sugar intake. High sugar consumption has been linked to cognitive decline and impaired memory.

6. Hydration:

- **Explanation:** The alkaline diet emphasizes water-rich foods like fruits and vegetables, contributing to hydration. Proper hydration supports cognitive function and mental clarity.

7. Antioxidant-Rich Foods:

- **Explanation:** Alkaline foods, especially colorful fruits and vegetables, are rich in antioxidants. Antioxidants help protect brain cells from oxidative stress and inflammation.

8. Balanced Nutrient Intake:

- **Explanation:** The diet encourages a balance of macronutrients, including carbohydrates, proteins, and healthy fats. Balanced nutrition provides the energy needed for optimal brain function.

9. Brain-Boosting Herbs and Spices:

- **Explanation:** Many herbs and spices used in alkaline cooking, such as turmeric, ginger, and rosemary, contain compounds that may support cognitive function and brain health.

10. Moderate Caffeine Consumption:

- **Explanation:** While not specifically emphasized in the alkaline diet, moderate caffeine intake from sources like green tea may provide a natural boost to alertness and cognitive function.

11. Mindful Eating:

- **Explanation:** The diet encourages mindful eating, which can support digestion and nutrient absorption. Proper nutrient absorption is crucial for delivering essential nutrients to the brain.

Lifestyle Practices for Optimal Brain Function

Optimal brain function is influenced not only by diet and herbs but also by lifestyle choices. Adopting specific practices that support brain health can contribute to enhanced cognitive function, memory, and overall well-being. Here's a detailed exploration of lifestyle practices that promote optimal brain function:

1. Regular Physical Exercise:

- **Explanation:** Engaging in regular physical activity improves blood flow to the brain, promotes the growth of new neurons, and enhances cognitive function. Aerobic exercises like walking, jogging, and swimming have been linked to improved memory and attention.

2. Mental Stimulation:

- **Explanation:** Keep your brain active by engaging in mentally stimulating activities. Puzzles, crosswords, chess, learning a new instrument, and engaging in creative projects challenge your brain and support cognitive function.

3. Adequate Sleep:

- **Explanation:** Prioritize getting 7-9 hours of quality sleep each night. Sleep is essential for memory consolidation, cognitive restoration, and overall brain health.

4. Stress Management:

- **Explanation:** Chronic stress can negatively impact cognitive function. Practice stress reduction techniques such as meditation, deep breathing, mindfulness, and relaxation exercises to promote mental clarity.

5. Social Engagement:

- **Explanation:** Maintaining social connections and engaging in meaningful interactions can stimulate brain activity and support cognitive health. Social engagement also helps reduce the risk of cognitive decline.

6. Healthy Relationships:

- **Explanation:** Cultivate healthy relationships that provide emotional support and meaningful connections. Positive social interactions have been shown to enhance brain health and overall well-being.

7. Mindfulness and Meditation:

- **Explanation:** Practicing mindfulness and meditation can improve attention, reduce anxiety, and enhance cognitive function. These practices promote relaxation and a clear state of mind.

8. Balanced Stress Hormones:

- **Explanation:** Keep stress hormones like cortisol in check through healthy lifestyle choices. Balanced hormones support brain health and cognitive function.

9. Continuous Learning:

- **Explanation:** Lifelong learning challenges your brain and promotes neuroplasticity, allowing your brain to adapt and develop new connections.

10. Healthy Relationships:

- **Explanation:** Cultivate meaningful relationships that provide emotional support and promote cognitive engagement. Positive social interactions contribute to brain health.

11. Regular Cognitive Assessments:

- **Explanation:** Consider engaging in cognitive assessments or brain training apps to track your cognitive performance over time.

12. Hydration:

- **Explanation:** Stay properly hydrated by drinking adequate water throughout the day. Dehydration can impair cognitive function.

13. Time Management:

- **Explanation:** Efficient time management reduces stress and helps you allocate time for work, relaxation, and activities that support brain health.

14. Limit Screen Time:

- **Explanation:** While technology has its benefits, excessive screen time can negatively impact cognitive function. Set limits on screen use to promote real-world interactions.

15. Creative Expression:

- **Explanation:** Engage in creative activities like art, music, writing, or crafting. Creative expression stimulates different areas of the brain and supports cognitive flexibility.

Book 19: Joint Freedom: Dr. Sebi's Natural Solutions for Joint Health

Joint Health: Common Issues and Causes

Joint health is vital for maintaining mobility, flexibility, and overall well-being. Joints are the connections between bones that allow movement and provide structural support. However, various factors can contribute to joint issues that affect millions of people worldwide. This chapter delves into the common joint issues and their underlying causes:

1. Osteoarthritis:

- **Explanation:** Osteoarthritis is the most prevalent form of arthritis, especially among older adults. It occurs when the protective cartilage that cushions the ends of bones wears down over time, leading to pain, swelling, and decreased joint function.
- **Causes:** Age is a significant factor, as cartilage naturally degenerates over time. Joint injuries, overuse, genetics, obesity, and poor joint alignment can contribute to osteoarthritis.

2. Rheumatoid Arthritis:

- **Explanation:** Rheumatoid arthritis is an autoimmune disorder that affects the joints. The immune system mistakenly attacks the synovium, the lining of the membranes that surround the joints, leading to inflammation and joint damage.
- **Causes:** The exact cause of rheumatoid arthritis is unknown, but genetic and environmental factors play a role. Smoking and certain infections may increase the risk.

3. Gout:

- **Explanation:** Gout is a form of arthritis caused by the buildup of uric acid crystals in the joints. It commonly affects the big toe, causing severe pain, swelling, and redness.
- **Causes:** Gout is often linked to diet and lifestyle factors. Consuming foods high in purines, excessive alcohol consumption, obesity, and genetic predisposition can contribute to gout.

4. Bursitis:

- **Explanation:** Bursitis is the inflammation of the bursae, small fluid-filled sacs that cushion the bones, tendons, and muscles near joints. It causes pain and restricted movement.

- **Causes:** Repetitive motions, joint overuse, injury, and certain medical conditions can lead to bursitis. It commonly affects the shoulder, elbow, hip, and knee.

5. Tendinitis:

- **Explanation:** Tendinitis is the inflammation of tendons, which connect muscles to bones. It can cause pain, stiffness, and reduced range of motion in the affected joint.
- **Causes:** Overuse, repetitive motions, poor posture, and age-related wear and tear can contribute to tendinitis. It commonly affects the shoulders, elbows, wrists, and heels.

6. Lupus Arthritis:

- **Explanation:** Lupus is an autoimmune disease that can affect various parts of the body, including the joints. Lupus arthritis causes joint pain, stiffness, and inflammation.
- **Causes:** The underlying cause of lupus is an overactive immune system that attacks healthy tissues. Genetic factors and environmental triggers may play a role.

7. Ankylosing Spondylitis:

- **Explanation:** Ankylosing spondylitis is a type of inflammatory arthritis that primarily affects the spine. It leads to stiffness, pain, and limited mobility in the spine and other joints.
- **Causes:** Genetics and immune system factors are believed to contribute to ankylosing spondylitis. It's more common in individuals with a family history of the condition.

Dr. Sebi's Herbal Support for Healthy Joints

Dr. Sebi, a renowned herbalist, advocated for a natural approach to health and wellness, including joint health. He believed that using specific herbs and natural remedies could support the body's healing processes and promote healthy joints. While individual experiences may vary, here's an explanation of some of the herbs and practices Dr. Sebi recommended for maintaining healthy joints:

1. Burdock Root:

- **Explanation:** Burdock root is known for its anti-inflammatory properties and potential to alleviate joint discomfort. It is believed to support detoxification and help the body eliminate waste, contributing to joint health.

2. Devil's Claw:

- **Explanation:** Devil's claw is traditionally used to address joint pain and inflammation. It contains compounds that may help reduce discomfort and improve mobility.

3. Nettle Leaf:

- **Explanation:** Nettle leaf is rich in nutrients and antioxidants. It's believed to have anti-inflammatory effects that could contribute to joint health by reducing inflammation.

4. Chaparral:

- **Explanation:** Chaparral is believed to possess anti-inflammatory and antioxidant properties. It has been traditionally used to support the body's natural healing processes and promote joint comfort.

5. Horsetail:

- **Explanation:** Horsetail is a plant rich in minerals like silica, which is essential for maintaining healthy connective tissues, including joints.

6. Bromide Plus Powder:

- **Explanation:** This herbal powder is a blend of sea moss and bladderwrack. It's believed to be rich in minerals that support joint health and overall wellness.

7. Dr. Sebi's Cell Food:

- **Explanation:** This herbal tonic is designed to nourish and revitalize the body. It contains a combination of herbs that Dr. Sebi believed could promote overall health, including joint health.

8. Hydrate with Natural Beverages:

- **Explanation:** Dr. Sebi recommended hydrating the body with natural, alkaline beverages like herbal teas, water, and fresh juices. Staying hydrated is important for maintaining joint health and overall well-being.

9. Alkaline Diet:

- **Explanation:** Dr. Sebi's approach also emphasizes the importance of an alkaline diet, rich in plant-based foods. Consuming alkaline foods is believed to support the body's natural healing processes, potentially benefiting joint health.

10. Detoxification:

- **Explanation:** Dr. Sebi's approach includes detoxifying the body to remove accumulated toxins. This cleansing process is believed to support joint health and overall vitality.

The Alkaline Diet for Joint Comfort

.kaline diet, inspired by Dr. Sebi's principles, emphasizes consuming foods that promote an .aline pH in the body. Proponents of this diet believe that it can contribute to overall health and well-being, including joint comfort. While scientific research on the alkaline diet's direct impact on joint health is limited, the diet's emphasis on plant-based, nutrient-rich foods aligns with general recommendations for promoting joint comfort. Here's an in-depth explanation of the alkaline diet's potential role in supporting joint health:

1. Plant-Based Foods:

Explanation: The alkaline diet encourages the consumption of fruits, vegetables, legumes, nuts, and seeds. These foods are rich in antioxidants, vitamins, and minerals that may support joint health by reducing inflammation and oxidative stress.

2. Anti-Inflammatory Benefits:

Explanation: Many foods promoted in the alkaline diet have anti-inflammatory properties, which could be beneficial for reducing joint inflammation and discomfort. Leafy greens, berries, turmeric, ginger, and other alkaline foods may contribute to this effect.

3. Balanced pH Levels:

Explanation: The diet aims to balance the body's pH levels by reducing the consumption of acidic foods like processed meats, dairy, and refined sugars. An alkaline environment may theoretically support joint health by reducing inflammation and creating an environment less conducive to inflammation-related discomfort.

4. Hydration:

Explanation: The alkaline diet promotes hydration through alkaline beverages like water and herbal teas. Staying hydrated is important for maintaining joint health, as proper hydration supports joint lubrication and function.

5. Reduced Processed Foods:

Explanation: The diet discourages processed and refined foods, which are often high in unhealthy fats, sugars, and additives. Avoiding these foods may help reduce the risk of inflammation-related joint discomfort.

6. Omega-3 Fatty Acids:

Explanation: The alkaline diet includes foods rich in omega-3 fatty acids, such as flaxseeds, chia seeds, walnuts, and certain leafy greens. Omega-3s have anti-inflammatory properties that can benefit joint health.

7. Magnesium-Rich Foods:

Explanation: Many alkaline foods are also good sources of magnesium, a mineral that supports muscle and joint relaxation. Magnesium-rich foods include leafy greens, nuts, seeds, and whole grains.

8. Avoiding Acidic Foods:

Explanation: The alkaline diet recommends minimizing or avoiding acidic foods, such as red meat, processed foods, and sugary snacks. These foods are believed to contribute to an inflammatory environment that could affect joint health.

9. Moderation and Balance:

Explanation: The diet emphasizes moderation and balance, which are key principles for overall health. A balanced diet supports optimal weight management, reducing the strain on joints and potentially alleviating discomfort.

Lifestyle Strategies for Joint Flexibility

Maintaining joint flexibility is crucial for overall mobility, comfort, and quality of life. A combination of healthy lifestyle strategies can help promote joint flexibility and reduce the risk of joint discomfort. Here's an in-depth explanation of lifestyle strategies that contribute to joint flexibility:

1. Regular Physical Activity:

- **Explanation:** Engaging in regular exercise helps keep joints mobile and flexible. Low-impact activities like walking, swimming, cycling, and yoga are especially beneficial for promoting joint flexibility without putting excessive strain on them.

2. Stretching and Range-of-Motion Exercises:

- **Explanation:** Incorporate gentle stretching and range-of-motion exercises into your routine. Stretching helps improve flexibility, reduce muscle tension, and maintain joint mobility.

3. Strength Training:

- **Explanation:** Building muscle strength supports joint stability and function. Focus on exercises that target the muscles around the joints, helping to provide support and reducing strain on the joints themselves.

4. Joint-Specific Exercises:

- **Explanation:** Some exercises are specifically designed to improve joint flexibility. For example, shoulder circles, hip circles, ankle circles, and wrist rotations can help maintain mobility in these joints.

5. Warm-Up and Cool-Down:

- **Explanation:** Before engaging in physical activity, warm up your muscles and joints with gentle movements and stretches. Afterward, cool down with stretches to maintain flexibility and prevent stiffness.

6. Maintain a Healthy Weight:

- **Explanation:** Excess weight can place additional stress on joints, leading to discomfort and reduced flexibility. Maintaining a healthy weight through a balanced diet and regular exercise supports joint health.

7. Hydration:

- **Explanation:** Staying hydrated supports joint lubrication and flexibility. Proper hydration helps maintain the synovial fluid that cushions and nourishes the joints.

8. Ergonomic Practices:

- **Explanation:** Ensure that your work environment is ergonomically designed to prevent strain on joints. Maintain proper posture while sitting, standing, and lifting to reduce the risk of joint discomfort.

9. Mindful Movement:

- **Explanation:** Practice mindfulness during movement to avoid overexertion or improper technique. Listen to your body and avoid pushing yourself beyond your limits.

10. Massage and Foam Rolling:

- **Explanation:** Regular massage and foam rolling can help release muscle tension, improve circulation, and maintain joint flexibility.

11. Quality Sleep:

- **Explanation:** Sleep is essential for tissue repair and overall well-being. Adequate sleep supports joint health by allowing the body to recover and regenerate.

12. Stress Management:

- **Explanation:** Chronic stress can contribute to muscle tension and joint discomfort. Practice stress-reduction techniques like meditation, deep breathing, and relaxation exercises.

13. Avoid Prolonged Inactivity:

- **Explanation:** Prolonged sitting or inactivity can lead to joint stiffness. Incorporate movement breaks throughout the day to keep joints limber.

Embracing Active Living: A Path to Pain-Free Joints

Embracing an active lifestyle is a key component of maintaining pain-free joints and overall well-being. Incorporating regular physical activity, healthy habits, and a positive mindset can significantly contribute to joint comfort and mobility. Here's an in-depth explanation of how embracing active living can lead to pain-free joints:

1. Regular Exercise:

- **Explanation:** Engaging in regular physical activity helps improve joint flexibility, strength, and overall function. Cardiovascular exercises, strength training, and flexibility routines contribute to maintaining healthy joints.

2. Low-Impact Activities:

- **Explanation:** Choose low-impact activities like walking, swimming, cycling, and yoga. These activities reduce the strain on joints while providing cardiovascular benefits and promoting joint comfort.

3. Maintain a Healthy Weight:

- **Explanation:** Excess weight can put additional stress on joints, leading to discomfort and reduced mobility. Achieving and maintaining a healthy weight through a balanced diet and exercise helps alleviate joint strain.

4. Balanced Nutrition:

- **Explanation:** A diet rich in nutrients, antioxidants, and anti-inflammatory foods supports joint health. Foods like fruits, vegetables, whole grains, lean proteins, and healthy fats contribute to pain-free joints.

5. Stay Hydrated:

- **Explanation:** Proper hydration supports joint lubrication and overall function. Drinking adequate water throughout the day helps maintain joint comfort and flexibility.

6. Proper Posture:

- **Explanation:** Maintain good posture while sitting, standing, and walking. Proper alignment reduces the strain on joints and supports overall musculoskeletal health.

7. Mind-Body Practices:

- **Explanation:** Practices like yoga, tai chi, and Pilates focus on mindful movement, balance, and flexibility. These practices enhance joint comfort, reduce muscle tension, and promote relaxation.

8. Quality Sleep:

- **Explanation:** Adequate sleep is essential for joint recovery and overall health. Sleep supports tissue repair, reduces inflammation, and contributes to pain relief.

9. Stress Management:

- **Explanation:** Chronic stress can exacerbate joint discomfort. Practice stress-reduction techniques like meditation, deep breathing, and spending time in nature to promote relaxation.

10. Listen to Your Body:

- **Explanation:** Pay attention to your body's signals. If you experience joint discomfort or pain, modify your activities or seek medical advice to prevent further strain.

11. Set Realistic Goals:

- **Explanation:** Set achievable fitness goals that align with your current abilities and needs. Gradual progression helps prevent overexertion and reduces the risk of joint discomfort.

12. Social Engagement:

- **Explanation:** Engaging in physical activities with friends, family, or fitness groups can enhance motivation and make staying active enjoyable.

13. Cultivate a Positive Mindset:

- **Explanation:** A positive attitude plays a role in maintaining an active lifestyle. Focus on the benefits of physical activity for joint health and overall well-being.

14. Regular Check-ups:

- **Explanation:** Regular visits to a healthcare professional help monitor joint health and address any concerns or discomfort promptly.

Book 20: Dr. Sebi's Alkaline Kitchen: Mouthwatering Plant-Based Recipes

Dr. Sebi's Alkaline Breakfast Creations

Dr. Sebi's dietary philosophy emphasizes consuming foods that promote an alkaline environment in the body. This approach aims to support overall health and well-being by focusing on plant-based, nutrient-rich foods. Breakfast is an important meal that sets the tone for the day, and Dr. Sebi's alkaline breakfast creations prioritize foods that align with his principles. Here's an in-depth explanation of some of Dr. Sebi's alkaline breakfast options:

1. Green Smoothie:

- **Explanation:** A green smoothie made with alkaline fruits like kiwi, green apple, and avocado, along with nutrient-rich greens like kale, spinach, and watercress. Blend these ingredients with alkaline water or herbal teas to create a refreshing and nutritious breakfast option.

2. Chia Seed Pudding:

- **Explanation:** Prepare a chia seed pudding using alkaline ingredients like chia seeds, unsweetened almond milk, and a touch of natural sweeteners like dates or stevia. You can top the pudding with sliced alkaline fruits like berries and kiwi.

3. Alkaline Oatmeal:

- **Explanation:** Create an alkaline oatmeal by using gluten-free oats, almond milk, and chopped alkaline fruits such as bananas and berries. Flavor it with natural spices like cinnamon and nutmeg, and sweeten with dates or agave syrup.

4. Quinoa Breakfast Bowl:

- **Explanation:** Cook quinoa in alkaline vegetable broth and top it with sautéed alkaline vegetables like bell peppers, zucchini, and spinach. Drizzle with cold-pressed olive oil and sprinkle with fresh herbs.

5. Plantain Pancakes:

- **Explanation:** Make pancakes using plantain flour or ripe plantains blended with almond milk, flaxseeds, and a pinch of sea salt. Serve these pancakes with fresh berries or an alkaline fruit compote.

6. Alkaline Smoothie Bowl:

- **Explanation:** Prepare a thick smoothie using alkaline fruits like mango, papaya, and berries. Pour the smoothie into a bowl and top it with chopped alkaline fruits, nuts, seeds, and a drizzle of almond butter.

7. Avocado Toast:

- **Explanation:** Spread mashed avocado on sprouted whole-grain bread or alkaline-friendly bread. Top with sliced tomatoes, cucumbers, and a sprinkle of sea salt and black pepper.

8. Fresh Fruit Salad:

- **Explanation:** Create a vibrant fruit salad using a variety of alkaline fruits like melons, berries, citrus fruits, and kiwi. Add fresh mint leaves for extra flavor.

9. Alkaline Breakfast Burrito:

- **Explanation:** Fill a sprouted whole-grain tortilla with sautéed alkaline vegetables, black beans, and avocado slices. Roll it up and enjoy a savory breakfast option.

10. Herbal Tea Infusions:

- **Explanation:** Start your day with herbal tea infusions using alkaline herbs like dandelion, nettle, or chamomile. These teas can be enjoyed alongside your alkaline breakfast.

Wholesome Alkaline Lunch Delights

Dr. Sebi's alkaline dietary principles emphasize consuming plant-based, nutrient-rich foods to promote an alkaline environment in the body. Lunch is an opportunity to nourish your body with vibrant ingredients that support your well-being. Here's an in-depth explanation of some of Dr. Sebi's wholesome alkaline lunch options:

1. Alkaline Veggie Stir-Fry:

Explanation: Sauté a variety of alkaline vegetables such as bell peppers, broccoli, cauliflower, zucchini, and mushrooms in cold-pressed olive oil or coconut oil. Flavor with alkaline herbs and spices like thyme, oregano, and garlic. Serve over quinoa or brown rice.

2. Stuffed Bell Peppers:

Explanation: Prepare stuffed bell peppers using a mixture of cooked quinoa, sautéed alkaline vegetables, and black beans. Top with a tomato sauce made from alkaline tomatoes, onions, and herbs.

3. Lentil Soup:

Explanation: Create a hearty lentil soup using alkaline lentils, alkaline vegetables, and flavorful herbs. Use alkaline vegetable broth as the base and add a touch of sea salt and black pepper.

4. Avocado and Chickpea Salad:

Explanation: Combine chopped avocado, cooked chickpeas, diced cucumbers, tomatoes, red onions, and fresh herbs. Dress the salad with a simple dressing made from lemon juice, cold-pressed olive oil, and alkaline spices.

5. Alkaline Wrap:

Explanation: Fill a sprouted whole-grain tortilla with hummus, sliced alkaline vegetables, avocado, and leafy greens. Roll it up for a convenient and nutritious alkaline wrap.

6. Cauliflower Rice Bowl:

Explanation: Process cauliflower into "rice" and sauté it with alkaline vegetables, such as peas, carrots, and scallions. Flavor with alkaline-friendly seasonings and serve with a side of alkaline hummus.

7. Alkaline Sushi Roll:

Explanation: Create a sushi roll using nori sheets, alkaline vegetables like cucumber, bell peppers, and avocado, and quinoa or cauliflower rice. Serve with a side of alkaline-friendly soy sauce or tamari.

8. Alkaline Pasta Salad:

Explanation: Prepare a pasta salad using gluten-free pasta, chopped alkaline vegetables, olives, and a lemon-based dressing. Add fresh herbs like basil and parsley for extra flavor.

9. Alkaline Buddha Bowl:

Explanation: Assemble a colorful bowl with a variety of alkaline ingredients such as cooked quinoa, roasted sweet potatoes, sautéed greens, avocado slices, and a tahini-based dressing.

10. Vegetable Curry:

Explanation: Create a warming vegetable curry using alkaline vegetables, coconut milk, and aromatic spices like turmeric, cumin, and coriander. Serve with alkaline-friendly grains like millet or quinoa.

Nourishing Alkaline Snacks and Desserts

Dr. Sebi's alkaline dietary approach encourages the consumption of nutrient-rich, plant-based foods to support overall health and well-being. Snacks and desserts can also be aligned with his principles by incorporating alkaline ingredients. Here's an in-depth explanation of some nourishing alkaline snack and dessert options:

Nourishing Alkaline Snacks:

1. Alkaline Veggie Sticks with Hummus:

- **Explanation:** Slice alkaline vegetables like cucumbers, bell peppers, and celery into sticks. Pair them with homemade alkaline hummus for a satisfying and nutritious snack.

2. Alkaline Trail Mix:

- **Explanation:** Create a trail mix using alkaline nuts (such as almonds and walnuts), seeds (like pumpkin and sunflower seeds), and dried alkaline fruits (such as apricots and raisins).

3. Alkaline Fruit Salad:

- **Explanation:** Combine a variety of alkaline fruits like melons, berries, and citrus fruits. Add a sprinkle of chopped alkaline herbs like mint for extra flavor.

4. Seaweed Snacks:

- **Explanation:** Enjoy roasted or seasoned seaweed sheets as a crunchy and alkaline-rich snack. Seaweed is nutrient-dense and provides minerals like iodine.

5. Alkaline Energy Balls:

- **Explanation:** Blend dates, almonds, chia seeds, and a touch of alkaline spices in a food processor. Form the mixture into small balls for a convenient on-the-go snack.

Nourishing Alkaline Desserts:

1. Alkaline Fruit Sorbet:

- **Explanation:** Blend frozen alkaline fruits like mango, pineapple, or berries until smooth. Enjoy the naturally sweet and refreshing sorbet.

2. Alkaline Chia Pudding Parfait:

- **Explanation:** Layer chia seed pudding with sliced alkaline fruits and chopped alkaline nuts. Drizzle with a touch of raw honey or maple syrup if desired.

3. Alkaline Banana Ice Cream:

- **Explanation:** Freeze ripe bananas, then blend them until creamy. Add a splash of almond milk and vanilla extract for extra flavor. Top with chopped alkaline nuts.

4. Alkaline Oat Cookies:

- **Explanation:** Create cookies using mashed ripe bananas, gluten-free oats, chopped alkaline fruits, and a hint of alkaline-friendly sweeteners like date syrup.

5. Alkaline Berry Crumble:

- **Explanation:** Mix fresh alkaline berries with a crumble topping made from almond flour, chopped alkaline nuts, and a touch of alkaline sweetener. Bake until golden and bubbly.

6. Alkaline Chocolate Avocado Mousse:

- **Explanation:** Blend ripe avocado, raw cacao powder, a touch of almond milk, and a natural alkaline sweetener like stevia to create a rich and creamy dessert.

Satisfying Alkaline Dinner Delicacies

Dr. Sebi's alkaline dietary principles promote the consumption of plant-based, nutrient-rich foods to create an alkaline environment in the body. Dinner is an opportunity to enjoy satisfying and flavorful meals that support your well-being. Here's an in-depth explanation of some satisfying alkaline dinner options:

1. Alkaline Stir-Fried Tofu and Veggies:

- **Explanation:** Sauté tofu cubes and a variety of alkaline vegetables like bell peppers, broccoli, and carrots in cold-pressed olive oil or coconut oil. Season with alkaline herbs and spices for a flavorful dish.

2. Alkaline Lentil Stew:

- **Explanation:** Prepare a hearty lentil stew using alkaline lentils, alkaline vegetables, and a flavorful alkaline broth. Add aromatic herbs and spices like thyme and cumin for depth of flavor.

3. Alkaline Quinoa Salad:

- **Explanation:** Create a quinoa salad using cooked quinoa, diced alkaline vegetables, chopped herbs, and a lemon-based dressing. Add chickpeas or black beans for added protein.

4. Alkaline Veggie Burger:

- **Explanation:** Make veggie burgers using mashed alkaline vegetables like sweet potatoes, black beans, and quinoa. Serve them on alkaline-friendly buns or lettuce wraps.

5. Alkaline Ratatouille:

- **Explanation:** Prepare a classic ratatouille using alkaline vegetables like eggplant, zucchini, tomatoes, and bell peppers. Flavor with alkaline herbs like thyme and rosemary.

6. Alkaline Stuffed Portobello Mushrooms:

- **Explanation:** Fill portobello mushroom caps with a mixture of sautéed alkaline vegetables, quinoa, and chopped alkaline nuts. Bake until mushrooms are tender.

7. Alkaline Cauliflower Curry:

- **Explanation:** Create a flavorful cauliflower curry using alkaline-friendly spices like turmeric, cumin, and coriander. Add alkaline vegetables and serve over brown rice or quinoa.

8. Alkaline Zucchini Noodles with Pesto:

- **Explanation:** Spiralize zucchini to create noodles and toss them with homemade alkaline pesto made from fresh herbs, alkaline nuts, and cold-pressed olive oil.

9. Alkaline Portobello Fajitas:

- **Explanation:** Marinate sliced portobello mushrooms in an alkaline-friendly fajita marinade. Sauté with alkaline bell peppers and onions, and serve with alkaline-friendly tortillas.

10. Alkaline Lentil Loaf:

- **Explanation:** Prepare a hearty lentil loaf using alkaline lentils, sautéed alkaline vegetables, and gluten-free breadcrumbs. Top with a homemade alkaline tomato sauce.

Made in United States
Troutdale, OR
03/06/2024